GLUTEN FREE COOKBOOK

150 fast and easy recipes for busy people on a gluten free diet

Olivia J. Collins

Copyright © 2020 Olivia J.Collins

All rights reserved.

CONTENTS

Introduction — 1

Chapter 1: Recognize Gluten-Containing Foods — Pg 3

Chapter 2: Delicious Breakfast & Brunch Favorites — Pg 7

- *Avocado Breakfast Bowl*
- *Baby Spinach Omelet*
- *Bacon Cheddar Drop Biscuits*
- *Banana Coconut Baked Oatmeal – Vegan*
- *Chorizo Breakfast Skillet*
- *GF French Toast With Bacon-Infused Syrup*
- *Hash & Spinach Eggs*
- *Raspberry-Peach Crisp Overnight Oats*

Delicious Bagels
- *French Toast Bagel*
- *Garlic Coconut Flour Bagels*
- *Mozzarella Dough Bagels*
- *Onion Low-Carb Bagel*

Waffles
- *Belgian Style Coconut Flour Waffles*
- *Chocolate Waffles - Keto-Friendly*
- *Healthy Almond Flour Waffles*

Pancakes
- *Blueberry Pancakes*
- *Pumpkin Pancakes*

Muffins
- *Bacon Egg Muffins*
- *Banana Muffins*
- *Blackberry Lemon Muffins*
- *Blueberry Lemon Muffins*
- *Chocolate Zucchini Muffins - Sugar-Free*
- *Cinnamon Rhubarb Muffins*
- *Coconut Flour Zucchini Bread Muffins*
- *Pepperoni Pizza Muffins*

Chapter 3: Pizza & Salad Time   Pg 33

Delicious Pizza
- *Bacon - Mushroom & Blue Cheese Pie*
- *Beet & Leek Cassava Crust Pizza*
- *Cheeseburger Pie*
- *Keto Pizza Pockets*
- *Spiralized Sweet Potato Crust Veggie Pizza - Vegan & Paleo*

Pizza Gluten-Free Pie Crusts
- *Almond Flour Pizza Crust*
- *Cauliflower Pizza Crust*
- *Coconut Flour Pizza Crust*
- *Fat Head Pizza Dough - Egg & Gluten-Free*

Healthy Salads
- *Cauliflower & Egg Salad*
- *Frozen Fresh Fruit Salad*
- *Granny's Loaded Broccoli Salad*
- *Kale-Salmon Caesar Salad*
- *Lemon Basil Pasta Salad*

Mediterranean Salad

Pecan & Apple Salad

Pomegranate Avocado Salad

Russian Cucumber & Radish Salad

Salmon Salad

Spinach Salad With GF French Salad Dressing

Strawberry Avocado Salad With Feta & Arugula

Strawberry Cucumber Salad

Thai Fruit Salad

Salad Breadsticks

Chapter 4: Side & Vegetable Dishes & Soup — Pg 62

Apple Coleslaw

Asparagus With Mushrooms & Hazelnuts

Baked Sweet Potatoes

Barbecue Fries

Broccoli Breadsticks

Cauli Mac 'N' Cheese

Cauliflower Rice

Creamy Potato Salad With Bacon

Crispy Tortilla-Crusted Zucchini - Dairy-Free

Ethiopian Cabbage

Green Beans With Pecans - Bacon & Blue Cheese

Holiday Cranberries With Apples & Brandy

Maple-Glazed Carrots

Provolone Grilled Eggplant

Roasted Asparagus With Olive Vinaigrette

- *Roasted Broccoli*
- *Roasted Butternut Squash With Mustard Vinaigrette*
- *Roasted Cauliflower With Tahini Sauce*
- *Sautééd Chard & Cashews*
- *Slow-Cooked Baked Beans*

Delicious Soup
- *Cream of Broccoli Soup*
- *Delicious Egg Drop Soup*
- *Fall Lamb & Veggie Stew*
- *Gazpacho Chilled Soup*
- *Italian Beef Soup*
- *Jambalaya Soup*
- *Sweet Corn - Kielbasa & Potato Soup*

Chapter 5: Chicken Specialties   Pg 92

- *Almond & Artichoke Stuffed Chicken Breasts*
- *Bacon Chicken Cutlets With Sweet Potato Mash*
- *Braised Chicken Thighs With Winter Vegetables*
- *Crispy Baked Chicken Fingers*
- *5 Cheese Mac & Cheese With Broccoli & Chicken*
- *Grilled Chicken With Warm Quinoa Salad & Carrots*
- *Lemon Pepper & Rosemary Rubbed Chicken*
- *Roasted Chicken With Fennel & Lemons*
- *Spatchcocked Chicken With Tomatoes*
- *Tandoori Chicken Drumsticks With Cilantro-Shallot Relish*
- *Tangy Chicken Cacciatore - Slow Cooked*

Yogurt Chicken Kebabs With Tomato Salad

Chapter 6: Pork Favorites Pg 107

Apple & Onion Slow-Cooked Pulled Pork

Carolina BBQ Pork Chops

Coconut Curry Pork Meatballs

Crispy Oven-Fried Pork Chops

Crockpot Pork Chops & Herb Gravy

Garlic Pot Roast

Instant Pot Ribs

1-Pan Ranch Pork Chops With Crispy Potatoes

Parmesan-Crusted Oven-Baked Pork Chops

Pork Or Lamb Pilaf With Raisins & Apricots

Pork Tenderloin With Onions & Peppers

Smothered Pork Chops

Chapter 7: Seafood Specialties Pg 123

Chettinad Crab Masala

Ginger Garlic Paste

Coconut Shrimp

Fish Fry With Shallots & Coconut

Flounder With Orange Coconut Oil

GF Crab Cakes

GF Lobster Cakes

Grilled Salmon

Lemon-Olive Oil Pasta With Tuna

Roasted Shrimp

Seafood Crepes

Seared Chilean Sea Bass

Shrimp - Asparagus & Quinoa Stir Fry

Chapter 8: Beef Favorites　　　　　　　　　Pg 139

Beef & Bean Casserole

Beef & Broccoli Stir Fry

Beef Stroganoff

Beef Taco Bowls

Taco Seasoning - For One Pound of Beef

Cheeseburger Casserole

Crunchy Taco Hamburger Helper

Mexican Quinoa & Beef - Slow-Cooked

Mini Philly Cheesesteak Meatloaves

Pepper Steak - Slow Cooker

Chapter 9: Snacks & Tasty Appetizers　　Pg 151

Bacon-Wrapped Figs

Bacon-Wrapped Jalapeno Poppers

Buffalo Quinoa Bites

Cheesy Mashed Potato Balls

Espinacas a la Catalana

Macho Nachos

Spinach Balls

Spinach & Artichoke Risotto Balls

Thai Mini Shrimp Lettuce Wraps

Tuna Spring Rolls

Vegan Avocado Boats

Chapter 10: Delicious Desserts   Pg 164

Almond Flour Cupcakes With Raspberry Frosting

Blueberry - Coconut Flour Scones

Carrot Cake

Chocolate Chip GF Mug Cake

Cinnamon Bread

Sugar-Free Donuts

Cookies

Almond Flour Cookies With Walnuts & Cranberries

Chocolate Zucchini Cookies

Coconut Chocolate Chip Cookies

Coconut Flour Cranberry Orange Cookies

Coconut Macaroons

Peanut Butter Blossoms - Sugar-Free

Quick & Easy Mug Cakes

Blueberry Mug Cake

Chocolate Brownie Mug Cake

Coconut Flour Pumpkin Mug Cake

Vanilla Berry Mug Cake

Conclusion

Introduction

Congratulations on purchasing *Gluten Free Cookbook* (also available in e-book). Thank you for adding it to your favorite recipes to assist you with your gluten-free (GF) alternatives for cooking and baking. Each segment is loaded with valuable information for you to carry throughout your gluten-free challenge. You will surely find a few items you did not realize contained the gluten demon. Gluten is the generic name for particular proteins found in the common cereal grains, including barley, rye, wheat, and their by-products.

I began this journey upon the recommendation of friends who had tried gluten-free options; I was sold on the prospects the way of cooking provided to them. So, I had to try it. In the process, I decided to share the wealth of my discovery! Please use the guidelines and delicious recipes with your friends and family for a delightful response! All of the recipes have been tested by many people.

These are just a few reasons you will enjoy the benefits of using the gluten-free recipes:

- Symptoms & complications with health-related issues are relieved.
- Promotes a healthier weight loss option
- Improves your cholesterol levels
- Helps with your digestive health and better bowel movements
- Improves the health of individuals who have arthritis or irritable bowel syndrome
- Could decrease the intake of refined or processed foods
- Increased energy levels

- You will now eat more foods that will contain more antioxidants, vitamins, and minerals.

Let's Begin!

CHAPTER 1: RECOGNIZE GLUTEN-CONTAINING FOODS

First, let's see how you can enjoy naturally-gluten-free foods. A few of the grains, flours, or starches that might be part of your gluten-free diet include the following:

- Gluten-free flours: Corn, soy, rice, potato, and bean flours
- Buckwheat
- Corn: Cornmeal, grits, and polenta labeled gluten-free
- Rice and wild rice
- Amaranth
- Arrowroot
- Flax
- Hominy (corn)
- Quinoa
- Millet
- Soy
- Sorghum
- Tapioca - cassava root

Fresh Naturally- GF Foods Allowed

Include many of these as part of a healthy diet:

- Lean, non-processed meats, fish and poultry
- Fruits & Vegetables
- Eggs
- Beans, legumes, seeds, and nuts (in their natural, unprocessed forms)
- Most low-fat dairy products

Foods That May Contain Gluten:

Read the labels to discover any items that contain wheat, barley, rye, and even oats in some cases.

While oats are naturally gluten-free, they may be contaminated during production with barley, wheat, or rye. Oats and oat products labeled gluten-free have not been cross-contaminated. Some people with celiac disease, however, cannot tolerate the gluten-free-labeled oats.

These are several wheat varieties to remove from your diet:

- Spelt
- Durum
- Emmer
- Einkorn
- Kamut

Wheat flours have different names based on how the wheat is milled or the flour is processed. All of the following flours have gluten:

- Graham flour - a coarse whole-wheat flour
- Self-rising flour - known as phosphate flour
- Enriched flour with added minerals and vitamins
- Farina - typically milled wheat is used in hot cereals
- Semolina - the part of milled wheat used in pasta and couscous
- Pasta - Ravioli, gnocchi, and dumplings

Be Aware of These Products:

- Noodles: Egg noodles, ramen, soba (some are made with only a percentage of buckwheat flour). (Note: Mung bean and rice noodles are free of gluten.)

- Granola: Be aware that many are made with regular - not gluten-free oats.

- Cereal: Rice puffs and corn flakes often contain malt extract/flavoring.

- Pastries & Bread: Naan, croissants, rolls, naan, flatbreads, pita, cornbread, donuts, potato bread, etc.

- Flour tortillas are another item to consider for their GF components.

- Panko breadcrumbs and other coatings/breading mixes.
- Gravies & Sauces: Traditional soy sauce, cream sauces made with a roux; some will use wheat flour for thickening sauces and gravy.
- Anything else that uses "wheat flour" as an ingredient

Read the Labels for These:

- Potato chips – Look for wheat starch or malt vinegar.
- Soup – cream-based soups frequently will use flour as a thickener. Barley is also an ingredient used in many processed soups.
- Meat substitutes made with seitan/wheat gluten include imitation seafood or veggie burgers. Tofu is gluten-free, but steer clear of soy sauce marinades.
- Soy Sauce: Use tamari made without wheat, which is gluten-free.
- Brown rice syrup – may be made with barley enzymes.
- Eggs served at restaurants – Some restaurants may add pancake batter in scrambled eggs and omelets, but solo, eggs are gluten-free.
- Pre-seasoned meats & processed lunch meats
- Of course, candy and candy bars

Reconsider the Spices - Sauces & Condiments

Even though most spices are *naturally* gluten-free, flavor enhancers, emulsifiers, and stabilizers may have been added. Some common gluten-containing ingredients can include malt, modified food starch, wheat flour, and maltodextrin.

Gluten-Free Baking Soda: When it comes to leavening, gluten-free recipes often need a little extra help—common gluten replacers simply aren't as elastic as regular gluten. Baking powder comes in two varieties; single-acting and double-acting. When engaging in gluten-free baking, you need to choose the double-acting baking powder. Here's the difference:

- *Double-Acting*: A chemical reaction takes place when the wet ingredients meet the powder. When it bakes, the product contains a second "high-heat" acid that is triggered by heat. This results in a higher, lighter texture.

- *Single-Acting*: When mixed with the wet ingredients that contain an acid, the baking powder begins its chemical reaction right away. The batter must go into the oven to bake immediately.

Let's get started on your new way of living!

CHAPTER 2: DELICIOUS BREAKFAST & BRUNCH FAVORITES

Avocado Breakfast Bowl

Yields Provided: 2
Total Time: 25-30 minutes

Ingredients Required:

- Water (.5 cup)
- Red quinoa (.25 cup)
- Olive oil (1.5 tsp.)
- Eggs (2)
- Black pepper & salt (1 pinch/as desired)
- Seasoned salt (.25 tsp.)
- Avocado (1 diced)
- Crumbled feta cheese (2 tbsp.)

Preparation Technique:

1. Toss the quinoa, salt, and water into a rice cooker. Set the timer for 15 minutes.
2. Warm oil in a skillet using the medium temperature setting. Cook the eggs, pepper, and seasoned salt.
3. Mix the eggs and quinoa. Top them off with a portion of the feta and avocado.

Baby Spinach Omelet

Yields Provided: 1
Total Time: 15 minutes

Ingredients Required:

- Eggs (2)
- Baby spinach leaves (1 cup)
- Onion powder (.25 tsp.)
- Grated parmesan cheese (1 tbsp. + .5 tsp.)
- Ground nutmeg (⅛ tsp.)
- Black pepper & salt (to your liking)

Preparation Technique:

1. Whisk the eggs and stir in the spinach, parmesan, pepper, salt, nutmeg, and onion powder.
2. Prepare a skillet using a cooking oil spray. Cook them for about three minutes, until partially cooked.
3. Flip them over with a spatula and continue cooking for another two to three minutes.
4. Lower the heat and simmer on low until it is done (2-3 min.). Serve immediately.

Bacon Cheddar Drop Biscuits

Yields Provided: 10
Total Time: 25 minutes

Ingredients Required:

- Almond flour (1.5 cups)
- Onion powder (1 tsp.)
- Baking powder (1 tbsp.)
- Garlic salt (1 tsp.)
- Baking soda (.5 tsp.)
- Dried parsley (1 tbsp.)
- Bacon (4 slices)
- Eggs (2)
- Sour cream (.5 cup)
- Bacon grease melted (1 tbsp.)
- Shredded cheddar cheese (1/3 cup)
- Shredded smoky bacon cheddar cheese (1/3 cup)
- Melted grass-fed butter (3 tbsp.)
- Swerve confectioners or powdered erythritol (.5 tsp.)

Preparation Technique:

1. Set the oven temperature in advance to 425° Fahrenheit.
2. Prepare a baking tin with a layer of baking paper.
3. Cook and crumble the bacon.
4. Add the baking powder, flour, onion powder, baking soda, and garlic salt into a mixing container using a fork or whisk.
5. Combine the eggs in with the melted butter, bacon grease, bacon, parsley, sour cream.
6. Fold the cheese and combine everything.
7. Scoop the biscuit mixture onto the prepared pan.
8. Bake them for 11 to 15 minutes.

Banana Coconut Baked Oatmeal – Vegan

Yields Provided: 2-3
Total Time: 30 minutes

Ingredients Required:

- Ground flaxseed (1 tbsp.)
- Water (3 tbsp.)
- Gluten-free rolled oats (1 cup)
- Unsweetened shredded coconut (2 tbsp.)
- Ground cinnamon (.25 tsp.)
- Nutmeg (1/8 tsp.)
- Baking powder (.25 tsp.)
- Coconut milk beverage from the carton, not the can (1 cup)
- Mashed ripe banana (.33 cup/about 1 medium)
- Pure vanilla extract (.25 tsp.)
- Also Needed: Ramekins (3)

Preparation Technique:

1. Warm the oven to reach 350° Fahrenheit. Spritz the ramekins with a cooking oil spray.
2. Whisk the flaxseed meal and three tablespoons of warm water. Wait for about five minutes.
3. Combine the shredded coconut, oats, nutmeg, cinnamon, and baking powder.
4. Whisk the coconut milk, vanilla extract, and mashed banana into the bowl with the flaxseed mixture.
5. Pour the dry fixings into the wet and stir until incorporated. Fill the ramekins and garnish with banana slices.
6. Bake until the oatmeal is puffed and set (20 min.) to serve right away.

Chorizo Breakfast Skillet

Yields Provided: 2
Total Time: 20 minutes

Ingredients Required:

- Olive oil (2 tsp.)
- Small onion (1)
- Chorizo cold cuts (6 slices)
- Cherry tomatoes (.5 cup)
- Sun-dried tomatoes (3)
- Eggs (4)
- Fresh basil (1 handful - slivered)

Preparation Technique:

1. Quarter the cold cuts and cut the cherry tomatoes into halves.
2. Warm oil in a skillet using the medium temperature setting.
3. Cut the onion in half and slice it. Toss it in the pan to sauté for about two minutes.
4. Mix in the chorizo, in a single layer, and cook it for two to three minutes.
5. Add the cherry tomatoes with the cut side down. Sauté them for two to three minutes.
6. Chop and fold in the sun-dried tomatoes and combine all of the fixings together. Use a spoon to make four mini craters in the four corners of the pan and crack four eggs (one into each hole), and sprinkle with the pepper and salt.
7. Continue cooking until the eggs are set. Serve with fresh basil.

GF French Toast with Bacon-Infused Syrup

Yields Provided: 4
Total Time: 5 minutes

Ingredients Required:

- Gluten-free bread (8 slices)
- Large eggs (3)
- Milk or dairy substitute (.5 cup)
- Vanilla (1.25 tsp.)
- Dark brown sugar (.25 cup)
- GF cornstarch (2 tbsp.)
- GF baking powder (1 tsp.)
- Salt (big pinch)
- Canola oil (1 tbsp.)
- Unsalted butter (2 tbsp.)

The Syrup:
- Bacon (2 slices)
- Water (.33 cup)
- Granulated sugar (.5 cup)
- Salt (1 pinch)
- Packed dark brown sugar (.5 cup)
- Vanilla (1.5 tsp.)

Preparation Technique:

1. Warm the oven at 350° Fahrenheit. Place eight slices of bread on a rack and bake them for approximately five minutes. Remove it and let it cool.
2. Cook the bacon until it is crispy. Cool and crumble for later.
3. In a flat dish, whisk the eggs, milk, vanilla, dark brown sugar, cornstarch, baking powder, and salt to remove all lumps.
4. Warm the oil and butter in a frying pan using the med-high temperature setting.
5. Dip the sliced bread into the batter, flipping once. Carefully transfer them to the frying pan. Cook them for

three to five minutes on each side. Lower the burner setting as needed.
6. Make the Syrup: Add one slice of crumbled bacon and the rest of the fixings in a large microwave-safe bowl. Reserve the second slice of bacon for the garnish. Whisk the syrup thoroughly.
7. Microwave the syrup on high for 45 seconds. Stir well. Return the dish to the microwave for 60 seconds. Stir and serve the toast warm with the bacon-infused syrup.

Hash & Spinach Eggs

Yields Provided: 4
Total Time: 35-40 minutes

Ingredients Required:

- Russet potatoes (3 medium)
- Olive oil (2 tbsp.)
- Small onion (1)
- Fresh spinach (1 cup)
- Garlic powder (.5 tsp.)
- Large eggs (4)
- Freshly cracked black pepper & salt (.25 tsp. each)

Preparation Technique:

1. Thoroughly scrub the potatoes and dot them using a fork. Pop them into the microwave for eight minutes or so until they're tender.
2. Roughly chop the potatoes (.5-inch bits) and toss them into a skillet with oil using the med-high temperature setting.
3. Chop the spinach and onion, and mince the garlic. Sauté them for about five to six minutes.
4. Press the spinach and hash into the pan. Make four "wells" in the center and add an egg to each one. Sprinkle them with the pepper and salt.
5. Place a lid on the pan and cook for about ten minutes until it's as desired and serve.

Raspberry-Peach Crisp Overnight Oats

Yields Provided: 2 parfaits
Total Time: 5 minutes

Ingredients Required:

- Vanilla Greek yogurt (12 oz.)
- GF raw old-fashioned oats (2/3 cup)
- Milk - any type (.25 cup)
- Optional: Chia seeds (2 tsp.)
- Vanilla (1 tsp.)
- Chopped peaches (2)
- Raspberries (6 oz.)
- Sliced almonds (.25 cup)

Preparation Technique:

1. In a large mixing container, combine the vanilla, chia seeds, milk, yogurt, and oats.
2. Scoop a fourth of the mixture into the jars with the peaches, berries, and one tablespoon of the almonds.
3. Repeat the layer and close the lids.
4. You can store them in the fridge for two to three days.

Delicious Bagels

French Toast Bagel

Yields Provided: 6 bagels
Total Time: 25 minutes

Ingredients Required:

- Melted butter (1/3 cup)
- Eggs (6)
- Cinnamon (1 tbsp.)
- Sugar-free vanilla extract (2 tsp.)
- Stevia glycerite (5-10 drops) or Swerve sweetener (1 to 1.5 tbsp.)
- Maple extract (1 tsp.)
- Salt (.5 tsp.)
- Sifted coconut flour (.5 cup)
- Xanthan gum or guar gum (.5 tsp. or optional)
- Baking powder (.5 tsp.)

Preparation Technique:

1. Set the oven temperature at 400° Fahrenheit. Lightly grease a donut pan.
2. Blend the eggs with the cinnamon, vanilla extract, maple extract, stevia, salt, and butter.
3. Whisk the coconut flour with the baking powder and guar/xanthan gum.
4. Combine everything and spoon it into the pan. Bake the bagels for 15 minutes.

Garlic Coconut Flour Bagels

Yields Provided: 6
Total Time: 35 minutes

Ingredients Required:

- Melted butter (1/3 cup)
- Sifted coconut flour (.5 cup)
- Optional: Guar gum or xanthan gum (2 tsp.)
- Eggs (6)
- Salt (.5 tsp.)
- Garlic powder (1.5 tsp.)
- Baking powder (.5 tsp.)

Preparation Technique:

1. Set the oven at 400° Fahrenheit.
2. Lightly grease a donut pan.
3. Blend the eggs, butter, salt, and garlic powder.
4. Combine coconut flour with baking powder and guar or xanthan gum.
5. Whisk the coconut flour mixture into the batter until there are no lumps.
6. Scoop it into the pan. Set a timer to bake for 15 minutes.
7. Wait for it to cool on a wire rack for 10-15 minutes. Transfer the bagels from the pan to cool or serve.

Mozzarella Dough Bagels

Yields Provided: 6
Total Time: 30-35 minutes

Ingredients Required:

- Mozzarella cheese (1.75 cups)
- Almond meal (.75 cup)
- Cream cheese (2 tbsp. - full- fat)
- Egg (1 medium)
- Baking powder (1 tsp.)
- Salt (1 pinch)

Preparation Technique:

1. Combine the shredded mozzarella cheese with the cream cheese and almond meal in a microwaveable bowl. Cook for one minute.
2. Stir the mixture and continue using the high setting for another 30 seconds.
3. Whisk the egg, baking powder, salt, and any other flavorings.
4. Portion the dough into six segments. Roll into balls and then into cylinder shapes.
5. Fold the ends together to form the bagels.
6. Arrange the bagels on a cookie tin and sprinkle with a few of the sesame seeds.
7. Bake at 425° Fahrenheit until golden brown (about 15 min.).

Onion Low-Carb Bagel

Yields Provided: 6
Total Time: 35-40 minutes

Ingredients Required:
- Flaxseed meal (3 tbsp.)
- Coconut flour (2 tbsp.)
- Baking powder (.5 tsp.)
- Eggs (4 separated)
- Dried minced onion (1 tsp.)

Preparation Technique:
1. Set the oven at 325° Fahrenheit.
2. Spray the donut baking pan with a spritz of cooking oil.
3. Combine the flax meal with the baking powder, coconut flour, and onion.
4. Mix the egg whites until foamy using an electric mixer.
5. Beat the yolks and combine the fixings.
6. Let the batter rest for about five to ten minutes to thicken.
7. Spoon into the donut mold. Sprinkle with additional dried onion to your liking.
8. Bake for 30 minutes. Allow cooling in the oven.

Waffles

Belgian Style Coconut Flour Waffles

Yields Provided: 4
Total Time: 10 minutes

Ingredients Required:
- Melted butter or ghee (4 tbsp.)
- Eggs (6)
- Salt (.5 tsp.)
- Baking powder (.5 tsp.)
- Coconut flour (1/3 cup)
- *Optional:* SweetLeaf stevia drops (1/8 tsp.)

Preparation Technique:
1. In a blender, mix the butter and eggs until incorporated.
2. Pour in the salt, stevia, and baking powder. Blend to combine.
3. Fold in the flour and let it rest to thicken (5 min.)
4. Pour in small amounts of water as needed to thin the batter.
5. Prepare in the waffle maker and serve.

Chocolate Waffles - Keto-Friendly

Yields Provided: 5
Total Time: 15 minutes

Ingredients Required:

- Medium eggs (5 separated)
- Coconut flour (4 tbsp.)
- Unsweetened cocoa (.25 cups)
- Swerve granulated sweetener of choice (4 tbsp. or more - as desired)
- Baking powder (1 tsp.)
- Vanilla (2 tsp.)
- Full-fat milk or cream (3 tbsp.)
- Melted butter (1 stick)

Preparation Technique:

1. In one container, add the egg whites. Whisk for a few minutes until you have formed stiff peaks.
2. In another container, whisk the yolks with the cocoa, sweetener, coconut flour, and baking powder.
3. Melt the butter and add to the fixings, mixing well to a smooth consistency.
4. Pour in the milk and vanilla. Stir well.
5. Fold in using spoonfuls of the prepared egg whites.
6. Pour the mixture into a preheated waffle maker.
7. Prepare one at a time until each one is golden brown. Continue the process until all are done. Serve with a smile for only three net carbs.

Healthy Almond Flour Waffles

Yields Provided: 8 waffles
Total Time: 10-15 minutes

Ingredients Required:

- Almond flour sifted (1 cup+ more as needed)
- Salt (.25 tsp.)
- *Optional*: Xanthan gum (.25 tsp.)
- Baking powder (1.5 tsp.)
- Heavy cream (1 cup + a little water)
- Oil (2 tbsp.)
- Eggs (3)

Preparation Technique:

1. Sift or whisk the flour with the salt, baking powder, and xanthan gum.
2. Pour in the oil and eggs. Whisk until incorporated.
3. *Special Note*: You may not use the entire cup of liquid. Slowly add heavy cream until the desired batter thickness is achieved. Adjust with flour or water as needed.
4. Pour into the waffle maker to cook.

Pancakes

Blueberry Pancakes

Yields Provided: 10 cakes
Total Time: 10-12 minutes

Ingredients Required:

- Eggs (4 medium)
- Coconut cream (1 cup)
- Vanilla (2 tsp.)
- Coconut flour (.5 cup)
- Swerve granular sweetener/your choice (4 tbsp.)
- Salt (1 pinch or as desired)
- Baking powder (1 tsp.)
- Blueberries or berries of choice (.5 cups)

Preparation Technique:

1. In a mixing container, whisk the vanilla, eggs, and coconut cream and until smooth.
2. Stir in the dry fixings (coconut flour, baking powder, sweetener, and salt). Whisk well to remove all of the lumps.
3. Prepare a skillet using the medium temperature setting to heat the oil.
4. Scoop a large spoonful of batter into the frying pan. Toss several blueberries onto each pancake.
5. Prepare each one until the top of the pancake starts to show bubbles. Flip the pancake over and prepare until they're done.
6. You can serve with whipped coconut cream and more berries with a portion of chopped nuts as desired. Just be sure to add any additional carbs for the indulgence.

Pumpkin Pancakes

Yields Provided: 4/10-12 small cakes
Total Time: 10 minutes

Ingredients Required:

- Almond flour (1 cup)
- Cinnamon (2 tsp.)
- Ground ginger (.5 tsp.)
- Allspice (.25 tsp.)
- Ground cloves (.125 tsp.)
- Salt (1 pinch)
- Baking powder (.5 tsp.)
- Canned pumpkin (.25 cup)
- Oil (2 tbsp.)
- Almond milk - unsweet (.25 cup)
- Erythritol (1 tbsp.)
- Stevia glycerite (1/8 tsp.)
- Eggs (2)

Preparation Technique:

1. Sift or whisk the almond flour with the spices, baking powder, and salt.
2. Stir in the rest of the fixings until well mixed (omitting the egg whites). Whip the whites into a stiff peak and then fold into the batter.
3. Drop by heaping tablespoonfuls into the pan.
4. Use the medium heat setting, flipping each pancake once.

Muffins

Bacon Egg Muffins

Yields Provided: 12
Total Time: 40 minutes

Ingredients Required:

- Bacon (12 slices)
- Large eggs (12)
- Cheddar cheese (8 oz. grated)

Preparation Technique:

1. Set the oven to reach 400° Fahrenheit.
2. Place the bacon on wire racks over a rimmed baking pan.
3. Bake it for 10-12 minutes, removing before it's crispy.
4. Spray the muffin tins with non-stick spray if needed. Line each tin with bacon.
5. Whisk the eggs and stir in the grated cheese and portion into the tin.
6. Bake them for about 25 minutes at 350° Fahrenheit or until the eggs are set.
7. Remove the muffins from the tins and serve warm.

Banana Muffins

Yields Provided: 6
Total Time: 45 minutes

Ingredients Required:

- Coconut oil (.25 cup)
- Monk fruit - 30% extract (.25 tsp.)
- Stevia powder extract (.25 tsp.)
- Banana extract (2 tsp.)
- Vanilla extract (1 tsp.)
- Large eggs (3)
- Baking powder (1 tsp.)
- Coconut flour (.25 cup)
- Almond flour (.75 cup)
- Salt (.25 tsp.)
- Cinnamon (.5 tsp.)
- Mashed avocado (1 medium)
- Pecans (.5 cup chopped)
- *Also Needed*: 6-count muffin tin

Preparation Technique:

1. Leave the eggs out to become room temperature.
2. Heat the oven at 350° Fahrenheit.
3. Generously grease the muffin tin.
4. Whisk the coconut oil with stevia and monk fruit.
5. Whisk in the eggs and mix with the vanilla and banana extracts.
6. In another container, sift or whisk the coconut flour, baking powder, cinnamon, almond flour, and salt.
7. Blend into the coconut oil mixture and the mashed avocado.
8. Fold in the nuts, reserving two tablespoons to sprinkle on top.
9. Pour the batter into the molds and garnish with the nuts.
10. Bake the muffins for approximately 25 to 30 minutes.

Blackberry Lemon Muffins

Yields Provided: 12
Total Time: 40-45 minutes

Ingredients Required:

- Almond flour (2 cups)
- Sea salt (1/8 tsp.)
- GF aluminum-free baking powder (2 tsp.)
- Coconut flour (1 tbsp.)
- Heavy cream (.5 cup)
- Large eggs - at room temperature (2)
- Melted butter (.25 cup)
- Lemon juice (1 tbsp.) & zest (1 lemon)
- Pure vanilla extract (1 tsp.)
- Liquid stevia (12 drops)
- Fresh firm blackberries or cherries / don't thaw if frozen (1.5 cups)
- Chopped pecans (.5 cup)

Preparation Technique:

1. Heat the oven to reach 350° Fahrenheit.
2. Prepare a muffin pan with parchment baking paper liners.
3. Mix the baking powder, almond flour, and salt into a food processor.
4. Pour in the cream, eggs, lemon juice, butter, lemon zest, vanilla, and stevia. Blend until creamy.
5. Fold in the blackberries and pecans.
6. Empty the mixture into the muffin tins.
7. Bake them for 30 to 35 minutes.
8. Cool in the pan.
9. *Note:* If you do not have a food processor, use an electric mixer.

Blueberry Lemon Muffins

Yields Provided: 10
Total Time: 30-35 minutes

Ingredients Required:

- Super-fine almond flour (1.75 cups)
- Oat fiber (.25 cup)
- Fresh blueberries (.75 cup)
- Eggs (2)
- Sour cream (1/3 cup)
- Heavy cream (1/3 cup)
- Baking powder (2 tsp.)
- Swerve confectioners (.5 cup)
- Juice & zest (1 lemon)
- Vanilla extract (1 tsp.)
- Salt (1 pinch)

Preparation Technique:

1. Warm the oven before it's time to bake to reach 350° Fahrenheit.
2. Whisk the oat fiber, baking powder, salt, and almond flour in a mixing container. Place the mixture to the side for now.
3. In another container, add the wet fixings, including the swerve. Mix using a whisk or hand mixer.
4. Combine all of the components and gently fold in the blueberries.
5. Empty into paper or silicone cupcake liners.
6. Bake for 18 to 20 minutes. Test with a cake tester for doneness. Allow cooling before serving.

Chocolate Zucchini Muffins - Sugar-Free

Yields Provided: 12
Total Time: 45-50 minutes

Ingredients Required:

- Eggs (5)
- Erythritol low-carb sweetener (.75 cup)
- Coconut oil or Melted butter (.5 cup)
- Salt - omit if using salted butter (.5 tsp.)
- Cocoa powder - unsweetened (3 tbsp.)
- Vanilla extract (.75 cup)
- Shredded zucchini (1 cup)
- Almond flour (1 cup)
- Baking soda (.5 tsp.)
- Coconut flour (.5 cup)
- Baking powder (.5 tsp.)
- Cinnamon (.5 tsp.)
- *Also Needed*: 12-count muffin baking mold

Preparation Technique:

1. Set the oven temperature at 325° Fahrenheit.
2. Lightly spritz the muffin molds with some cooking oil spray.
3. Whisk the sweetener and butter or oil in a mixing container. Add in the eggs, vanilla, cocoa, and zucchini.
4. In another container, combine each of the fixings and add the batter to the prepared molds.
5. Bake the muffins for 25 to 30 minutes.
6. Transfer the muffins from the molds to cool on a wire rack.
7. Serve as desired.

Cinnamon Rhubarb Muffins

Yields Provided: 12
Total Time: 30-35 minutes

Ingredients Required:

- Almond flour (.75 cup)
- Coconut flour (.25 cup)
- GF Baking powder (1.5 tsp.)
- Swerve (.25 cup)
- Kosher salt (.25 tsp.)
- Cinnamon (1 tsp.)
- Baking soda (.25 tsp.)
- Sour cream (.5 cup)
- Melted unsalted butter (4 tbsp.)
- Large eggs (2)
- Vanilla extract (.5 tsp.)
- *Sweet Leaf* stevia drops (1/8 tsp.)
- Diced rhubarb (1 cup)
  The Topping:
- Low-carb sweetener or Swerve (1.5 tbsp.)
- Ground cinnamon (.25 tsp.)

Preparation Technique:

1. Set the oven temperature at 400° Fahrenheit.
2. Lightly grease a 12-count muffin pan.
3. Whisk the dry fixings (both types of flour, swerve, salt, baking powder, cinnamon, and baking soda).
4. In another container, mix the wet ingredients (sour cream, butter, eggs, vanilla, and stevia).
5. Combine everything and fold in the prepared rhubarb.
6. Dump into the muffin cups.
7. Meanwhile, sprinkle about ½ teaspoon of the sweetened cinnamon mix over each muffin and bake for about 20 minutes.
8. Cool in the pan for 10 to 15 minutes.
9. Serve warm. Refrigerate the leftovers.
10. Reheat in a toaster oven for 5 to 10 minutes as desired.

Coconut Flour Zucchini Bread Muffins

Yields Provided: 12
Total Time: 35 minutes

Ingredients Required:

- Large eggs (6)
- Coconut oil liquified (1/3 cup)
- Baking soda (.25 tsp.)
- Coconut flour (.5 cup)
- Low-carb sweetener (.5 cup or 3.5 tbsp. of Truvia)
- Salt (.5 tsp.)
- Ground cinnamon (1 tsp.)
- Shredded zucchini (1.5 cups)
- *Optional*: Chopped walnuts (.5 cup)

Preparation Technique:

1. Set the temperature in the oven at 350° Fahrenheit.
2. Combine the first seven ingredients until well blended.
3. Fold in the zucchini and walnuts.
4. Spoon the batter into greased muffin cups or paper liners.
5. Bake the muffins for 20-25 minutes or test with a cake tester to check for doneness.

Pepperoni Pizza Muffins

Yields Provided: 12
Total Time: 40-45 minutes

Ingredients Required:

- Asiago cheese shredded (.5 cup)
- Cream cheese (5 oz.)
- Coconut flour (.25 cup)
- Baking powder (1 tsp.)
- Almond flour (2/3 cup)
- Salt (.5 tsp.)
- Water (3 tbsp.)
- Eggs (5 beaten)
- Mini pepperoni (.5 cup or about 2 oz.)
- Mozzarella cheese - shredded and divided (1 cup)

Preparation Technique:

1. Heat the oven in advance to reach 400° Fahrenheit.
2. Spritz the muffin molds with some cooking oil spray.
3. Whisk the eggs. Combine the cream cheese with the grated Asiago cheese, both types of flour, salt, baking powder, water, and the egg.
4. Fold in .5 cup of the mozzarella and the pepperoni.
5. Fill muffin cups about half full.
6. Toss on the rest of the mozzarella cheese.
7. Bake until the muffins are firm and lightly browned (25 to 30 min.).
8. Enjoy it at room temperature, hot, or straight from the refrigerator.
9. Store the leftovers in the fridge.

CHAPTER 3: PIZZA & SALAD TIME

Delicious Pizza

Bacon - Mushroom & Blue Cheese Pie

Yields Provided: 10 slices
Total Time: 50-55 minutes

Ingredients Required:

- Super-fine almond flour (1.5 cups)
- Egg (1)
- Coconut flour (1 tbsp.)
- Salt & pepper (1 pinch)
- *Blue Cheese Bacon - Mushroom Pie Filling*
- Butter - for frying (2 tbsp.)
- Garlic cloves (2 crushed)
- Bacon (4 slices - diced)
- Mushrooms (0.8 lb. - quartered)
- Heavy cream (.5 cup)
- Blue cheese/ favorite cheese (3.5 oz.)
- Eggs (4 medium - lightly beaten)
- *Also Needed*: 9.5-inch pie/flan dish

Preparation Technique:

1. Combine all of the fixings using a fork. Grease the pan with a spritz of cooking oil spray.
2. Place the pie crust onto the prepared dish using a layer of parchment baking paper on top and smooth out the pie crust. Remove the top baking paper.
3. Poke holes over the base with a fork for even browning and to help prevent the base from rising with a bubble.
4. Bake the pie at 350º Fahrenheit for 15 minutes. Transfer to the countertop to slightly cool.

5. Prepare the filling. Warm the butter in a skillet. Gently fry the bacon, garlic, and mushrooms until softened, and the water has evaporated.
6. Remove from the heat to cool down.
7. Combine the lightly beaten eggs, heavy cream, and blue cheese. Pour over the mixture over the pie crust.
8. Place the bacon, garlic, and mushroom mixture evenly into the egg mixture.
9. Bake at 350° Fahrenheit for 20 to 30 minutes until cooked in the center, but do not overcook.

Beet & Leek Cassava Crust Pizza

Yields Provided: 2 pies
Total Time: 20 minutes

Ingredients Required:

The Dough:
- Cassava flour (1 cup)
- Arrowroot starch (.5 cup)
- Baking powder (2 tsp.)
- Olive oil (4 tsp.)
- Seltzer (1 cup)

The Sauce:
- Cooked beets (3 small)
- Italian Cipollini onions (2)
- Zest of 1 lemon
- Garlic (1 tsp.)
- Fresh parsley (1 tbsp.)
- Black pepper (.25 tsp.)
- Nutritional yeast (2 tbsp.)

The Toppings:
- Golden beet (1 large)
- Leek (white part - 1 large)
- Fresh tarragon (2 tsp.)
- Fresh parsley (2 tsp.)

Preparation Technique:

1. Slice the beet into ⅛-inch rounds. Slice the leek into thin rounds. Finely chop the tarragon and parsley. Mince the garlic.
2. Set the oven at 425° Fahrenheit.
3. Prepare the dough in a stand mixer or large mixing container.
4. Scoop out the dough ball and break it in half to roll into the pizza base using a rolling pin.
5. Bake the crust for about ten minutes.

6. Prepare the sauce by combining each of the fixings in a food processor until they're smooth.
7. Top the prebaked crust with the sauce, beets, leeks, and herbs.
8. Note: A traditional Italian onion has a flat - oval shape that ranges in diameter size from one to three inches.

Cheeseburger Pie

Yields Provided: 8 slices
Total Time: 40-45 minutes

Ingredients Required:

- Venison/ground beef burger (1 lb.)
- Onion (1 cup)
- Salt (.5 tsp.)
- Coconut flour (1/3 cup)
- Almond flour (3 tbsp.)
- Bak. powder (1 tsp.)
- Almond milk - unsweet (1 cup)
- Large eggs (4)
- Shredded cheese (1.5 cups)
- Optional: Tomato (1)

Preparation Technique:

1. Warm the oven to reach 400° Fahrenheit.
2. Chop the onions and toss them into the skillet with the meat. Simmer for about eight to ten minutes.
3. Spread the beef mixture into the pie plate. Lightly dust with the salt.
4. Whisk the coconut flour with the almond flour, baking powder, eggs, and milk. Add to the meat along with one cup of cheese on the top.
5. Set the timer and bake the pie for approximately 25 minutes.
6. When ready, garnish with the rest of the cheese and tomato if desired.
7. Bake an additional five minutes.

Keto Pizza Pockets

Yields Provided: 4
Total Time: 20 minutes

Ingredients Required:

- Pre-shredded/grated cheese mozzarella (1.75 cups)
- Almond flour (.75 cup)
- Full-fat cream cheese (2 tbsp.)
- Egg (1 medium)
- Salt (1 pinch or to taste)

Preparation Technique:

1. Combine the cream cheese, shredded cheese, and flour in a microwaveable bowl. Prepare it using the high power function for one minute.
2. Stir and continue cooking on high for another 30 seconds.
3. Whisk the egg and salt and mix gently with the rest of the fixings.
4. Prepare the dough by rolling it between two sheets of parchment baking paper. (Don't roll as thin as a thin pizza crust so it can hold the chosen fillings.)
5. Discard the top baking paper. Slice the dough into squares (the same size as your toasted sandwich maker).
6. Place one square on the bottom of the sandwich maker, add your choice of fillings.
7. Place another square of dough on the top and press the lid of the sandwich maker down.
8. Cook until they're golden brown or about three to five minutes.

Spiralized Sweet Potato Crust Veggie Pizza - Vegan & Paleo

Yields Provided: 1
Total Time: 15 minutes

Ingredients Required:

- Sweet potato (1 large)
- Baby radishes (3)
- Brussels sprouts (3 large)
- Bell peppers (3 large)
- Flax eggs (2 mixed with milled flaxseed (2 tbsp.) + Water (6 tbsp.)
- Nutritional yeast (1-2 tbsp.)

The Sauce:
- Unsalted tomato paste (2 tbsp.)
- Garlic (.5 tsp.)
- Black pepper (.25 tsp.)
- Dried oregano (1 tsp.)

Dried Spices (.5 tsp. of each)
- Onion powder
- Marjoram
- Basil

Preparation Technique:

1. Do the Prep: Spiralize the potato with a 3mm blade. Slice the radishes and prep the peppers into rings. Mince the garlic. Chop the sprouts into quarters. Prepare the flax eggs by mixing the flaxseed and water and let them rest.
2. Warm the oven at 450° Fahrenheit. Spritz a cast-iron skillet, 9-inch round baking dish, or baking sheet with a layer of parchment baking paper.
3. Gently combine the potato with the eggs (use your hands).
4. Combine the sauce fixings in a mixing container.

5. Scoop the spiralized potato in the center of the chosen pan to form a tight circle. Spoon in the sauce, veggies, and nutritional yeast.
6. Bake for 15 to 18 minutes and serve.

Pizza Gluten-Free Pie Crusts

Almond Flour Pizza Crust

Yields Provided: 8
Total Time: 25-30 minutes

Ingredients Required:

- Almond flour (1.5 cups)
- Grated parmesan cheese (.5 cup)
- Flax meal or Whole psyllium husks (1 tbsp.)
- Baking powder (.5 tsp.)
- Oregano (.5 tsp.)
- Basil (.5 tsp.)
- Garlic powder (.5 tsp.)
- Large eggs (2)
- Water (2 tbsp. or more if needed)
- Olive oil (1 tbsp.)

Preparation Technique:

1. Set the oven temperature at 375° Fahrenheit.
2. Whisk the almond flour with the parmesan cheese, basil, oregano, psyllium baking powder, and garlic powder.
3. In another dish, whisk the oil with the water and eggs. Pour the mixture into the dry components, adding more water if needed.
4. Shape the dough into a ball. Prepare between two layers of parchment baking paper. Roll it out and transfer to a pizza pan. Discard the top paper.
5. Bake until the crust is browned for about 20-25 minutes. Cool for about 15 minutes.
6. Flip the crust over in the pan. Discard the paper. Add the pizza sauce and chosen toppings.
7. Bake under the oven broiler to melt the cheese and fixings to your liking.

Cauliflower Pizza Crust

Yields Provided: 4
Total Time: 15 minutes

Ingredients Required:

- Riced cauliflower - cooked (1 cup)
- Egg (1)
- Shredded mozzarella cheese (1 cup)
- *Optional:* Spices- ex. parsley, oregano or fennel

Preparation Technique:

1. Warm the oven at 450° Fahrenheit.
2. Spritz a baking tin with a portion of cooking oil spray.
3. Mix the cauliflower with the mozzarella and egg.
4. Press into the pan.
5. Sprinkle with the chosen spices and garlic powder.
6. Bake for 12-15 minutes. Pour in the sauce, toppings, and cheese.
7. Crank the oven to broil and arrange the pizza on the rack until the cheese is melted.
8. You can freeze the pizza crusts can be frozen after the initial baking and to be used later.

Coconut Flour Pizza Crust

Yields Provided: 6
Total Time: 40-45 minutes

Ingredients Required:

- Coconut flour (1/3 cup)
- Parmesan cheese (.25 cup)
- Flaxseed meal or psyllium, or almond flour (2 tbsp.)
- Olive oil (1-2 tbsp.)
- Large eggs (4)
- Garlic powder (1 tsp.)
- Cream of tartar (.25 tsp.)
- Parsley (1 tsp.)
- Salt (.25 tsp.)
- Italian Seasoning Blend (1 tsp.)
- Mozzarella cheese (.75 cup)

Preparation Technique:

1. Warm the oven at 375° Fahrenheit. Spritz a pizza pan with cooking oil spray.
2. Place all of the fixings into a food processor except for the mozzarella cheese.
3. Fold in the mozzarella cheese and toss onto the prepared baking tray.
4. Bake it until browned or for about 20 to 25 minutes.
5. Slice into strips for breadsticks.
6. For pizza, pour on the sauce and toppings.
7. Bake it at 350° Fahrenheit for about 12 minutes.

Fat Head Pizza Dough - Egg & Gluten-Free

Yields Provided: 8
Total Time: minutes

Ingredients Required:

- Mozzarella cheese slices full fat (8 oz.)
- Grated parmesan cheese (2 tbsp.)
- Full-fat cream cheese (2 tbsp.)
- Almond flour (1/3 cup)
- Garlic powder (.5 tsp.)
- Salt (.5 tsp.)
- Psyllium husks either whole or ground (2 tbsp.)

Preparation Technique:

1. Finely chop and place the mozzarella in a microwaveable container. Cook until melted. (This took about 1.5 minutes.)
2. Let the cheese cool slightly. Mix with the cream cheese, almond flour, parmesan cheese, garlic powder, and salt. (Knead in with your hands.)
3. Add the psyllium, shape the dough into a ball, and roll out as flat as you can on parchment paper, pizza stone, or a silicone mat.
4. Shape the dough as needed and bake at 425° Fahrenheit for about 15-20 minutes.
5. Flip the crust and bake for about five more minutes until browned.
6. Add the sauce, cheese, and other toppings. Bake it for about five more minutes.

Healthy Salads

Cauliflower & Egg Salad

Yields Provided: 1
Total Time: 5-10 minutes

Ingredients Required:

- Hard-boiled eggs (2)
- Cauliflower (1 cup)
- Celery (1 stalk)
- Red onion (1)
- Dill pickles (1 large)
- Yellow mustard (1 tbsp.)

Preparation Technique:

1. Dice the pickle and eggs. Chop the cauliflower.
2. Combine each of the fixings to serve fresh!
3. Chill and use later if desired.

Frozen Fresh Fruit Salad

Yields Provided: 12-18 servings
Total Time: 15 minutes

Ingredients Required:

- Chilled heavy whipping cream (2 cups)
- Cream cheese (8 oz. pkg.)
- Milk (.25 cup)
- Confectioners sugar (.33 cup)
- Crushed pineapple (12-16 oz. can as desired)
- Fruit cocktail (2-14-oz. cans)
- Chopped red maraschino cherries 1 (10-oz. jar)
- Dash of salt
- Pecans (1 cup - chopped)

Preparation Technique:

1. Whip the cream into stiff peaks using an electric mixer.
2. Combine the milk, confectioner's sugar, and softened cream cheese in another mixing container.
3. Prepare the fruits into a colander and drain thoroughly. Toss them in with the cream cheese mixture. Add in the whipped cream.
4. Lightly spray the baking dish with a spritz of cooking oil spray.
5. Add the delicious mixture to the pan and freeze it until firm.
6. Remove it from the freezer 15 minutes before serving time.
7. Slice it into squares to serve.

Granny's Loaded Broccoli Salad

Yields Provided: 8
Total Time: 1.25-1.5 hours

Ingredients Required:

- Frozen peas (2 cups)
- Cauliflower (1 lb.)
- Broccoli (1 lb.)
- Bacon (4 strips)
- GF mayonnaise (.5 cup)
- Plain yogurt or sour cream (.5 cup)
- Sugar (.5 tbsp.)
- Sharp cheddar (1 cup)
- Salt (.5 tsp.)

Preparation Technique:

1. Prepare the cauliflower and broccoli, chopping the stems, and cutting flowerets into bite-sized pieces. Dice the cheese into ½-inch pieces.
2. Fill a pot with four quarts of water and one tablespoon of salt.
3. Once boiling, add the peas and cook for one minute. Transfer to a colander to drain.
4. Use two batches in the same water to boil the cauliflower for three minutes, remove, and add the broccoli to cook for three minutes. Drain them under cold water to cool the veggies
5. Fry the bacon in a skillet using the medium temperature setting until it is crispy. Drain it on a paper-towel-lined platter.
6. Once cooled, combine the rest of the fixings and toss thoroughly.
7. Place a cover on the container and pop it into the refrigerator for about 60 minutes before serving. It is also delicious if made the day before dinner time.

Kale-Salmon Caesar Salad

Yields Provided: 2
Total Time: 5-6 minutes

Ingredients Required:

- Chopped-stemmed kale (5 cups
- Drained salmon (6 oz. can)
- GF Caesar salad dressing (2/3 cup)
- Shredded parmesan cheese (.5 cup)
- Freshly cracked black pepper & salt (.25 tsp. each)

Preparation Technique:

1. Drain the salmon and toss the fixings in a large salad bowl.
2. Serve immediately for freshness!

Lemon Basil Pasta Salad

Yields Provided: 6
Total Time: 30 minutes

Ingredients Required:

- GF pasta - ex. - orzo, elbow, shell (12 oz.)
- Olive oil (.25 cup)
- Balsamic vinegar (.25 cup)
- Lemon zest (1 tbsp. - 1 lemon)
- Juice from 1 lemon (about .25 cup)
- Sour cream (1 heaping tbsp.)
- Garlic powder (.5 tsp.)
- Black pepper (as desired)
- Salt (1 tsp.)
- Tomatoes (3 lb.)
- Cucumber (1 large)
- Fresh basil leaves (.5 cup - packed)
- Mozzarella - bite-size pieces (8-oz.)

Preparation Technique:

1. Remove the seeds from the tomatoes and cucumber. Peel and chop them for the salad. Tear the basal to pieces and slice the mozzarella into bite-sized pieces.
2. Follow the directions of the package of pasta, and cook it al dente.
3. Whisk the salt, pepper, oil, vinegar, sour cream, garlic powder, and lemon juice and zest.
4. Stir in the mozzarella, basil, cucumber, and tomatoes.
5. Drain the pasta (do not rinse) and combine all of the fixings.
6. Serve it now or chill for later!

Mediterranean Salad

Yields Provided: 3-5
Total Time: 5-8 minutes

Ingredients Required:

- Romaine lettuce (1 medium head)
- Tomatoes (3 small)
- Onion (1 small)
- Cucumber (1 medium)
- Green bell pepper (1 small)
- Radishes (6)
- Flat-leaf parsley (.5 cup)
- Avocado/olive oil (1/3 cup)
- Garlic clove (1)
- Lemon juice (3 tbsp.)
- Fresh mint (1 tsp.)
- Pepper and salt (as desired)

Preparation Technique:

1. Prep the veggies. Tear the lettuce to pieces. Thinly slice the radish, peppers, and cucumber. Slice the onion into rings. Dice/mince the garlic and tomatoes. Chop the parsley and mint.
2. Toss the radishes, onion, pepper, tomatoes, lettuce, and parsley in a large salad dish.
3. Whisk the oil, lemon juice, salt, garlic, mint, and pepper. Dump it over the salad to serve.

Pecan & Apple Salad

Yields Provided: 4-6
Total Time: 10 minutes

Ingredients Required:

- Mixed greens (6-8 cups)
- Red cabbage (¼ of 1 head)
- Apple (1)
- Pecans (.5 cup)
- Red onion (¼ of 1)
- Currants (.25 cup)
- Pumpkin seeds (.25 cup)
- Hemp seeds (.25 cup)
  The Dressing:
- Apple cider vinegar (1 tbsp.)
- Dijon mustard (1 tsp.)
- Olive oil (3 tbsp.)
- Black pepper & salt (to your liking)

Preparation Technique:

1. Do the prep. Thinly slice the cabbage and onion. Dice the apple and chop the pecans.
2. Toss each of the fixings into a large salad container.
3. Combine the dressing ingredients and whisk thoroughly.
4. Sprinkle the salad with dressing and serve.

Pomegranate Avocado Salad

Yields Provided: 1
Total Time: 5-6minutes

Ingredients Required:

- Spinach/Mixed greens/arugula/red leaf lettuce (1 cup)
- Ripe avocado (1)
- Pomegranate seeds (.5 cup)
- Pecan (.25 cup)
- Blackberries (.25 cup)
- Cherry tomatoes (.25 cup)

  Dressing - As Desired:
- Avocado/olive oil
- Salt
- Lemon juice

Preparation Technique:

1. Cut the avocado into ½-inch pieces and combine with the berries, pomegranates, tomatoes, pecans, and greens.
2. Whisk the dressing (oil, salt, juice) until thoroughly mixed and pour it over the salad to serve.

Russian Cucumber & Radish Salad

Yields Provided: 2-3
Total Time: 8-10 minutes

Ingredients Required:

- Medium Lebanese cucumbers (2)
- Radishes (6-8 small to medium)
- Spring (green) onions sliced thinly (2)
- Light sour cream (.5 cup)
- Fresh dill (2 tbsp.)
- Salt & pepper (as desired)

Preparation Technique:

1. Slice the cucumbers and radishes into thinly sliced rounds. Thinly slice the spring onions and chop the dill.
2. Combine each of the fixings and serve.

Salmon Salad

Yields Provided: 4
Total Time: 10 minutes

Ingredients Required:

- Pink salmon (2 cans)
- Bell pepper (half of 1)
- Celery (2 stalks)
- Red onion (.25 cup)
- Salt (1 tsp.)
- Avocado (.75 to 1 cup)
- To Serve: Salad greens or wrap
- Garnish: Everything But The Bagel Seasoning

Preparation Technique:

1. Drain the salmon into a mixing container and separate it.
2. Slice/dice the peppers, onion, and celery. Mash the avocado and combine it all with salt or any other desired spices.
3. Serve it over mixed greens of your choice.

Spinach Salad With GF French Salad Dressing

Yields Provided: 6 (The Salad)
The Dressing: 32 servings/1 pint
Total Time: 10 minutes

Ingredients Required:

- Spinach leaves (1 lb.)
- GF bacon (4 slices)
- Hard-boiled eggs (3)
- Red onions (1 cup)
- Mushrooms (1 cup)
- Optional: Smoked paprika (.25 tsp.)
  Gluten-Free Salad Dressing (1 recipe below)
- Extra-virgin olive oil (1 cup)
- Sugar (.5 to .75 cup or less if you like a less sweet dressing)
- Gluten-free ketchup (1/3 cup)
- Apple cider vinegar (.25 cup)
- Worcestershire sauce (1 tsp.)

Preparation Technique:

1. Rinse and dry the spinach and cook the bacon. Finely chop the eggs and thinly slice the mushrooms and onions.
2. Make the dressing by placing each of the fixings in a medium mixing container. Whisk it until the sugar is dissolved. Store it in a closed container in the fridge and use it as desired.

Strawberry Avocado Salad With Feta & Arugula

Yields Provided: 6
Total Time: 15 minutes

Ingredients Required:

The Vinaigrette:
- Olive oil (.5 cup)
- Dijon mustard (1 tbsp.)
- Vinegar preference - balsamic/red wine/white wine (3 tbsp.)
- Raw honey or maple syrup (1 tbsp.)

Optional: Chili flakes (.5 tsp./to taste)
- Sea salt (.5 tsp.)
- Black pepper (.25 tsp.)
- Optional: Garlic - pressed/minced (1)

The Salad
- Fresh arugula or baby spinach (6 packed cups)
- Strawberries - rinsed, hulled and halved (1 pint)
- Red onion (half of a small)
- Crumbled feta cheese (.75 cup)
- Roughly chopped pecans (2/3 cup)
- Avocados (2 ripe)

Preparation Technique:

1. Mince the garlic and thinly slice the onion. Rinse the berries, remove the ends as needed, and slice into halves. Rinse and spin the spinach. Peel, pit, and dice the avocados.
2. Combine the dressing fixings in a clean jar and add the salt and pepper as desired. Seal the top and shake it thoroughly. Set it aside until the salad is ready to serve.
3. Prepare the arugula/baby spinach in a salad dish.
4. Remove the green pieces from the berries and slice them into halves.

5. Thinly slice the onion and toss it into the bowl.
6. Dice and add the avocado, chopped pecans, and crumbled feta.
7. Add the dressing as desired and toss to serve.

Strawberry Cucumber Salad

Yields Provided: 4
Total Time: 10 minutes

Ingredients Required:

- Strawberries (2 cups)
- Cucumbers (2 large)
- Onion (half of 1 medium)
- Balsamic vinegar (.25 cup)
- Olive oil (2 tbsp.)
- Feta cheese (.5 cup)

Preparation Technique:

1. Slice the cucumbers, onion, and strawberries. Toss them with the oil and vinegar.
2. Crumble the feta and toss it over the salad. Omit the feta for a vegan option.

Thai Fruit Salad

Yields Provided: 6
Total Time: 15 minutes

Ingredients Required:

- Fresh/canned/frozen pineapple cubes (1 cup)
- Banana (1)
- Mango - frozen if fresh - ripe mangoes are not available (1 cup)
- Lychee fruit (if using canned, discard the liquid (1 cup)
- Star fruit (1)
- Strawberries (1-2 cups)
  For the Dressing:
- Coconut milk (.25 cup)
- Sugar (2-3 tbsp. or to taste)
- Fresh lime juice (1 tbsp.)

Preparation Technique:

1. Whisk each of the dressing components until the sugar is dissolved.
2. Prepare the fruit. Slice the banana. Peel and cube the mango and discard the liquid in the lychee fruit if it's canned. Peel and slice the star fruit.
3. Toss the ingredients well and scoop/pour the salad into a carved-out pineapple or serving dish as desired to serve.
4. Right before serving, garnish the salad with a star fruit slice and refrigerate until ready to serve.

Salad Breadsticks
Yields Provided: 16
Total Time: 25-30 minutes

Ingredients Required:

- Almond flour (1.5 cups)
- Psyllium husk powder (1 tbsp.)
- Baking powder (2 tsp.)
- Nutritional yeast (1 tbsp.)
- Dried basil (.5 tsp.)
- Garlic salt (1 tsp.)
- Dried parsley (2 tsp.)
- Shredded mozzarella cheese (2.5 cups)
- Cream cheese (3 oz.)
- Eggs (2)
- Grated parmesan cheese (2 tbsp.)
- Garlic cloves (2)
- Flavorless oil - as needed for prep
- Olive oil for brushing the tops

Preparation Technique:

1. Warm the oven before baking time to reach 400° Fahrenheit.
2. Prepare the garlic cloves with a press.
3. Place the mozzarella and cream cheese in a microwaveable container and set the timer to cook for one minute.
4. Mix in and whisk the almond flour, nutritional yeast, psyllium husk powder, oregano, garlic salt, parsley, basil, and baking powder in another container.
5. Whisk and mix in the eggs with the mozzarella, fresh garlic, and cream cheese.
6. Combine and add in the parmesan, then add in the dry fixings.
7. Divide the dough into eight pieces. Shape into logs and divide into sixteen breadsticks total.
8. Arrange them on a layer of parchment baking paper.
9. Bake it on the top rack of the oven (12 min.). Rotate the pan about halfway through the cooking cycle.

10. When the time is up, transfer to the countertop and lightly brush olive oil over the tops.
11. Bake them for an additional three minutes. Cool slightly before serving.

CHAPTER 4: VEGETABLE DISHES & SOUP

Apple Coleslaw

Yields Provided: 1-2
Total Time: 5-8 minutes

Ingredients Required:

- Cabbage - Multicolored (1 cup)
- Tart apple (1)
- Celery (1 stalk)
- Red pepper (1)
- Olive/avocado oil (.5 tsp.)
- Juice (1 lemon)
- Sea salt (1 dash)
- Optional: Raw honey (2 tbsp.)

Preparation Technique:

1. Chop each of the fixings (cabbage, apple, celery, and pepper).
2. Whisk the honey, juice, oil, and salt. Drizzle it over the slaw and toss.

Asparagus With Mushrooms & Hazelnuts

Yields Provided: 4
Total Time: 10-15 minutes

Ingredients Required:

- Fresh asparagus (1 lb.)
- Mushrooms (6 cups)
- Green onions (.5 cup.)
- Lemon juice (2 tbsp.)
- Coconut oil (2 tbsp.)
- Sea salt (.25 tsp.)
- Black pepper (as desired)
- Hazelnuts (2 tbsp.)

Preparation Technique:

1. Slice/chop the onions and mushrooms. Chop and toast the hazelnuts.
2. Whisk one tablespoon of the oil, juice, pepper, and salt.
3. Trim the ends from the asparagus and toss into a pan to steam for a few minutes.
4. Add the rest of the oil in a skillet using the high-temperature setting. Toss in the mushrooms and onions to sauté until softened (1-2 min.).
5. Fold in the asparagus to sauté another three minutes.
6. Transfer the pan to the countertop and slowly stir in the freshly squeezed juice.
7. Add the toasted nuts to serve.

Baked Sweet Potatoes

Yields Provided: 2
Total Time: 40-45 minutes

Ingredients Required:

- Sweet potatoes (2 medium)

Preparation Technique:

1. Warm the oven to reach 425° Fahrenheit.
2. Wash the potatoes and cut them into quarters.
3. Put them in a casserole dish with a lid.
4. Bake them until softened (about 40 min.).

Barbecue Fries

Yields Provided: 4
Total Time: 40 minutes

Ingredients Required:

- Olive oil (5 tbsp.)
- BBQ sauce (6 tbsp.)
- Hot pepper sauce (.5-1 tsp.)
- Black pepper (.5 tsp.)
- Optional: Paprika (.5 tsp.)
- Optional: Ground cumin (.25 tsp.)
- Russet/baking potatoes (2 lb.)
- For Serving: Optional: Sour cream
- Also Needed: Rimmed baking sheet

Preparation Technique:

1. Thoroughly scrub the potatoes.
2. Warm the oven to reach 450° Fahrenheit.
3. Spritz the baking tray with cooking oil.
4. Whisk the rest of the oil with the paprika, cumin, pepper, barbecue sauce, and hot pepper sauce.
5. Slice the potatoes (lengthwise) into eight to ten wedges. Toss them in the mixture and arrange them on the prepared pan.
6. Bake for 25-30 minutes - turning once until they are nicely browned.
7. Enjoy them with the sour cream for dipping.

Broccoli Breadsticks

Yields Provided: 3-4
Total Time: 35-40 minutes

Ingredients Required:

- Broccoli (4 cups/1 head)
- Nutritional yeast (3 tbsp.)
- Optional: Psyllium husk (1 tbsp.)
- Eggs (2 whole or a flax-gel replacement)
- Fresh basil (1 handful)
- Sea salt (.25 tsp.)
- Water (2 tbsp.)

Preparation Technique:

1. Warm the oven to reach 375° Fahrenheit.
2. Remove the tips of the broccoli stem and chop it into chunks. Toss it into a food processor to make the rice.
3. Add and pulse the basil, salt, psyllium husk, and nutritional yeast.
4. Combine the eggs, water, and broccoli mixture. Spread the dough over the sheet as desired.
5. Bake it until it's browned and the center is done to serve (30-35 min.).

Cauli Mac 'N' Cheese

Yields Provided: 6
Total Time: 25-30 minutes

Ingredients Required:

- Salt (as needed)
- Cauliflower (1 large head)
- Vegan butter (for the pan)
- Vegan heavy cream (1 cup)**
- Dijon mustard (2 tsp.)
- Vegan cream cheese (2 oz.)
- Shredded vegan cheddar (1.5 cups)
- Salt and pepper (to your liking)
- Nutritional yeast (1 tbsp.)
- Minced garlic (.5 tsp.)
- GF breadcrumbs (topping)

Optional Fixings: (.5-1 cup):
- Broccoli
- Vegan chicken
- Seitan
- Tempeh bacon
- Marinated tofu

Preparation Technique:

1. Set the oven at 375° Fahrenheit. Cut the cauliflower into small florets. Cut the cream cheese into chunks and shred the cheddar cheese.
2. Pour water and salt into a large pot and wait for it to boil.
3. Meanwhile, cover the baking dish with butter, or you can also use a high-heat oil.
4. Toss the cauliflower in the boiling water and cook until tender (5 min.). Dump it into a colander to drain and place it in a tea towel or a layer of paper towels. Add it to the baking dish.
5. Bring the heavy cream to a simmer in a saucepan. Whisk in the mustard and cream cheese.

6. Fold in and whisk one cup of the shredded cheese, pepper, salt, garlic, and nutritional yeast (1-2 min.).Pour it over the cauliflower and other desired fixings, stirring to combine.
7. Garnish it using the rest of the cheese and a layer of breadcrumbs. Bake until bubbly hot and browned to your liking (15 min.).
8. **Note: Make the heavy cream. Vegan dairy-free heavy cream = Plain soy milk (.5 cup) + 1 block of silken tofu (12-oz.). Blend in a blender until thick and creamy, and there are no more lumps.

Cauliflower Rice

Yields Provided: 2
Total Time: 10-15 minutes

Ingredients Required:

- Cauliflower (1 head)
- Coconut oil (2 tbsp.)
  Optional Seasonings – As Desired:
- Ground black pepper
- Ginger
- Garlic
- Sea salt

Preparation Technique:

1. Prep the cauliflower to a rice-like consistency in a food processor.
2. Sprinkle it using salt and pepper.
3. Prepare a skillet using the high-temperature setting to warm the oil.
4. Sauté the 'rice' and garnish as desired to serve.

Creamy Potato Salad With Bacon

Yields Provided: 8
Total Time: 30 minutes

Ingredients Required:

- Small red new potatoes (3 lb./24)
- Kosher salt (1 tsp. + .75 tsp.)
- Sliced bacon (8 pieces)
- Mayonnaise (.5 cup)
- Sour cream (.25 cup)
- White wine vinegar (3 tbsp.)
- Black pepper (.5 tsp.)
- Flat-leaf parsley (.5 cup)
- Celery (4 stalks)
- Fresh tarragon (.25 cup)

Preparation Technique:

1. Thinly slice the celery. Chop the parsley and tarragon. Set them to the side for now.
2. Prepare a pot of water with enough cold water to cover the potatoes. Add about one teaspoon of salt and wait for it to boil. Lower the temperature setting and simmer until tender (15-18 min.).
3. Drain the potatoes under cold water. When they are chilled slightly, slice them into quarters.
4. Prepare the bacon in a skillet using the medium temperature setting until it's crispy (6-8 min.). Drain them on a paper towel-lined platter. Wait for it to cool and crunch them to bits.
5. Whisk the pepper, ¾ teaspoon of salt, vinegar, sour cream, and mayo. Add the celery and potatoes, tossing to coat them thoroughly.
6. Chop and fold in the parsley, bacon, and tarragon before serving.

Crispy Tortilla-Crusted Zucchini – Dairy-Free

Yields Provided: 3-4
Total Time: 40-45 minutes

Ingredients Required:

- Zucchini (1 lb./about 3 medium-sized)
- Salt (.5 tsp. – divided)
- Jackson's Honest organic tortilla chips – Finely crushed (.75 cup)
- Almond flour/meal (.5 cup)
- Garlic powder (.25 tsp.)
- Large egg (1)

Preparation Technique:

1. Warm the oven to reach 375° Fahrenheit.
2. Slice the zucchini into halves (lengthwise) and slice again (horizontally) for four pieces and slice them into spears.
3. Sprinkle the spears with about ¼ teaspoon of salt and place them in a colander.
4. Mix the flour, chips, rest of the salt, and garlic powder in a shallow preparation pan.
5. Pat dry the zucchini and dredge them through the egg yolk, roll it in the chips – pressing to help the chips stick.
6. Arrange each of them on a baking pan to bake for 18 minutes. Switch the oven to broil (2-3 min.) until they're crispy.
7. Transfer to serving dish and serve.

Ethiopian Cabbage

Yields Provided: 5
Total Time: 1 hour 10 minutes

Ingredients Required:

- Olive oil (.5 cup)
- Carrots (4)
- Onion (1)
- Sea salt (1 tsp.)
- Black pepper (.5 tsp.)
- Ground turmeric (.25 tsp.)
- Ground cumin (.5 tsp.)
- Cabbage (½ of 1 head)
- Potatoes (5)

Preparation Technique:

1. Warm the oil in a skillet using the medium temperature setting.
2. Prep the veggies. Thinly slice the onion and carrots. Peel and slice the potatoes into one-inch cubes. Shred the cabbage.
3. Toss in the onion and carrots to sauté for about five minutes. Stir in the spices (cumin, turmeric, salt, and pepper), and cabbage.
4. Toss in the potatoes and cover to cook using the med-low temperature setting. Cook about 20-30 minutes until they are softened.
5. Serve when ready!

Green Beans With Pecans – Bacon & Blue Cheese

Yields Provided: 4
Total Time: 15 minutes

Ingredients Required:

- Green beans (1 lb.)
- Bacon (3 slices)
- Blue cheese (4 oz.)
- Candied pecans (.5 cup)
- Kosher salt and black pepper (.5 tsp. of each)

Preparation Technique:

1. Trim the tips from the beans and chop the pecans.
2. Prepare a large pot of water using the high-temperature setting.
3. When boiling, pour in the beans to simmer for three minutes.
4. Dump the beans into a colander to drain. Then, toss them in a container of ice water for three minutes to stop the cooking process.
5. Add the bacon to a large skillet (med-high temp) and fry for four to five minutes on each side.
6. Remove when they are crispy on a towel-lined plate to remove the fats.
7. Toss the beans into the pan drippings and sauté for two to three minutes over the med-high temperature setting.
8. Chop the bacon and toss all of the fixings together to serve.

Holiday Cranberries With Apples & Brandy

Yields Provided: 8
Total Time: 40 minutes

Ingredients Required:

- Cranberries (2 – 12 oz. bags/6 cups)
- Granny Smith apples (2 medium)
- Sugar (2 cups)
- Orange juice (.25 cup)
- Brandy (2 tbsp.)
- Also Needed: 4-quart oven-proof dish

Preparation Technique:

1. Peel, remove the core, and slice the apples into ½-inch cubes.
2. Set the oven to reach 375° Fahrenheit.
3. Combine the orange juice, cranberries, apples, sugar, and brandy. Toss in the baking dish and thoroughly mix it before covering with a layer of aluminum foil.
4. Bake it until the fruit is softened (40 min.). Remove from the oven and stir.
5. Serve it hot, chilled, or at room temperature.

Maple-Glazed Carrots

Yields Provided: Varies / 6-8
Total Time: 20-25 minutes

Ingredients Required:

- Water (1 cup)
- Carrots (2 lb.)
- Salt and black pepper (.5 tsp. each)
- Pure maple syrup (.25 cup)
- Unsalted butter (2 tbsp.)

Preparation Technique:

1. Peel and chop the carrots. Pour the water, salt, and carrots into a large skillet.
2. Once it's boiling, lower the temperature setting to low medium and cover for about eight minutes to cook until they are tender.
3. Toss the carrots into the pan with butter, syrup, and pepper.
4. Increase the heat setting to medium and stir for about five minutes. Serve it piping hot and thoroughly glazed.

Provolone Grilled Eggplant

Yields Provided: 8 as a first course/4 as a main course
Total Time: 45 minutes

Ingredients Required:

- Olive oil (3 tbsp.)
- Dried oregano (.25 tsp.)
- Balsamic vinegar (1.5 tbsp.)
- Eggplants (4 – cut in half lengthwise)
- Thick deli-style mild provolone (.5 lb.)
- Black pepper
- Kosher salt (.5 tsp.)
- Grilled salsa

Preparation Technique:

1. Whisk the oil, vinegar, and oregano. Brush the mixture over the cut sides of the eggplants and dust with pepper and salt.
2. Warm a gas grill using the high setting, lowering the temperature to medium after about 15 minutes. (If you are using charcoal, wait for the coals to burn until they are gray ash.)
3. Arrange the eggplants on the grill with the cut-side down until browned (5 min.). Turn them over and top each half with a provolone slice.
4. Grill until the cheese is bubbly (3 min.). Top with grilled salsa.

Roasted Asparagus With Olive Vinaigrette

Yields Provided: 4
Total Time: 15 minutes

Ingredients Required:

- Asparagus (2 bunches/2 lb.)
- Olive oil (3 tbsp.)
- Pitted kalamata olives (.5 cup)
- Flat-leaf parsley (2 tbsp.)
- Black pepper & kosher salt (.25 tsp./as needed)
- Red wine/sherry vinegar (1 tbsp.)
- Essential: Rimmed baking sheet

Preparation Technique:

1. Chop the olives and parsley after trimming the asparagus.
2. Set the oven to reach 450° Fahrenheit. Toss the asparagus with one tablespoon of the oil, pepper, and salt.
3. Cook them until they're tender – tossing one time (8-12 min.).
4. Mix the vinegar, parsley, olives, the rest of the oil (2 tbsp.), and ¼ teaspoon each pepper and salt. Spoon it over the asparagus and serve.

Roasted Broccoli

Yields Provided: 4
Total Time: 30-35 minutes

Ingredients Required:

- Broccoli florets (1 lb.)
- Olive oil (2 tbsp.)
- Black pepper and salt (1 tsp. of each)
- Freshly grated parmesan cheese (.25 cup)

Preparation Technique:

1. Set the oven to reach 350° Fahrenheit.
2. Chop the broccoli into bite-sized pieces and arrange them (single-layered) on a rimmed baking tray. Spritz them with oil, salt, and pepper.
3. Roast them for 25-30 minutes.
4. After the broccoli is tender, drizzle it with the fresh cheese, and serve.

Roasted Butternut Squash With Mustard Vinaigrette

Total Time: 1 hour 15 minutes
Yields Provided: 8

Ingredients Required:

- Butternut squash (3 small/2 lb. each)
- Shallots (8)
- Cider vinegar (1 tbsp.)
- Apple cider (1 cup)
- Kosher salt and black pepper (.75 tsp. of each + more as desired)
- Olive oil (4 tbsp.)
- Whole-grain mustard (1 tbsp.)
- Flat-leaf parsley (.25 cup – fresh)
- Also Needed: 2 large rimmed baking sheets.

Preparation Technique:

1. Heat the oven to 375° Fahrenheit.
2. Peel, remove the seeds, and slice the squash into ½-inch thick half-moons.
3. Slice the shallots into wedges and chop the parsley.
4. Divide the shallots and squash into the baking trays.
5. Toss the veggies with oil (2 tbsp.) and ½ teaspoon each of the pepper and salt. Roast them (single-layered) until golden brown and tender (50-55 min.).
6. Let the cider cook until it's reduced in volume to about ¼ of a cup (12-15 min.). Cool it for five minutes.
7. Whisk in the mustard, parsley, vinegar, the rest of the oil, black pepper, and salt to your liking.
8. Place the shallots and squash in your serving dish with a spritz of vinaigrette to serve.

Roasted Cauliflower With Tahini Sauce

Yields Provided: 6
Total Time: 40-45 minutes

Ingredients Required:

- Avocado or olive oil (.25 cup)
- Ground cumin (4 tsp.)
- Cauliflower (2 heads)
- Tahini (.5 cup)
- Black pepper & salt (as desired)
- Garlic cloves (3)
- Water (.5 cup)

Preparation Technique:

1. Prep the cauliflower by removing the core and chopping it into 1.5-inch florets. Mash the garlic into a paste and squeeze the lemon.
2. Roast the cauliflower in a 450° Fahrenheit oven for about 35 minutes.
3. Whisk the tahini, water, juice, and garlic with salt.
4. Serve the cauliflower chilled – or not – with the sauce.

Sautééd Chard & Cashews

Yields Provided: 2
Total Time: minutes

Ingredients Required:

- Swiss chard (1 bunch)
- Coconut oil (1 tbsp.)
- Cashews (.5 cup)
- Optional: Black pepper & sea salt

Preparation Technique:

1. Wash and remove the tough stems from the chard. Chop it into thin strips.
2. Use the medium temperature setting to heat a skillet with the oil.
3. Toss the chard and cashews into the skillet to sauté with the pepper and salt for one minute.
4. Serve it warm.

Slow-Cooked Baked Beans

Yields Provided: 12
Total Time: 1.5-3 hours

Ingredients Required:

- Small red beans (4 cans – 15 oz. each)
- Bacon (6 slices)
- Onion (1 cup)
- Green bell pepper (.5 cup)
- GF ketchup (1 cup)
- Packed brown sugar (.5 cup)
- GF mustard (2 tsp.)
- GF Maple syrup (2 tbsp.)
- Garlic powder (1.5 tsp.)
- Apple cider vinegar – ACV (1 tsp.)
- Salt and black pepper (.5 tsp.)

Preparation Technique:

1. Rinse and drain the beans. Finely chop the pepper and onion. Cook and crumble the bacon. Toss each of the fixings into the pot. Stir thoroughly.
2. Place the lid on the slow cooker and set the timer for 1.5 hours on high or three hours on low.
3. Note: Make it vegan by removing the bacon! Be sure to check the labels for gluten.

Delicious Soup

Cream of Broccoli Soup

Yields Provided: 4
Total Time: 10-12 minutes

Ingredients Required:

- Fresh broccoli (1.5 lb.)
- Water (2 cups)
- Tapioca flour (.5 cup) + Water (1 cup – cold)
- Pepper (as desired)
- Salt (.75 tsp.)
- Coconut cream (.5 cup)

Preparation Technique:

1. Steam/boil the broccoli until tender.
2. Pour the water and cream into a double boiler with the pepper, salt, and broccoli.
3. Mix the flour and water in a small container and pour it into the soup. Stir until thickened to serve.

Delicious Egg Drop Soup

Yields Provided: 4-6
Total Time: 5-7 minutes

Ingredients Required:

- Chicken broth (1.5 quarts)
- Tapioca flour (2 tbsp. + .25 cup cold water)
- Eggs (2)
- Scallions (2)

Preparation Technique:

1. Add the broth to a pot to heat. Once boiling, slowly mix in the tapioca mixture to thicken the broth.
2. Slightly whisk the eggs with a fork and lower the heat setting as you mix in the eggs. Turn off the heat.
3. Chop the scallions and add them to the top to serve.

Fall Lamb & Veggie Stew

Yields Provided: 6-8
Total Time: Varies – 7 hours 15 minutes

Ingredients Required:

- Lamb stew meat (2 lb.)
- Zucchini (1)
- Summer squash (1)
- Chopped tomatoes (2)
- Mushrooms (1 cup)
- Onions (1 cup)
- Bell peppers (.5 cup)
- A crushed clove of garlic (1)
- Salt (2 tsp.)
- Bay leaf (1)
- Thyme leaves (.5 tsp.)
- Chicken broth (2 cups)

Preparation Technique:

1. Chop/dice the veggies. Toss the lamb and veggies into a crockpot.
2. Combine the rest of the fixings and simmer for seven hours using the low-temperature setting.

Gazpacho Chilled Soup

Yields Provided: 4
Total Time: 20 minutes + chill time

Ingredients Required:

- Flaxseed meal (.5 cup)
- Tomatoes (4 cups)
- Bell peppers (1 green & 1 red)
- Cucumber (1)
- Garlic (2 cloves)
- Virgin olive/avocado oil (150 ml)
- Lemon juice (2 tbsp.)

Preparation Technique:

1. Peel the cucumber and dice it with the peppers and tomatoes. Mince the garlic. Mix in the oil and flax meal. Blend it until smooth.
2. Adjust the salt and lemon juice as preferred.
3. Pop it in the fridge to chill.
4. Serve the soup with a sprinkle of parsley, mint, black olives, or hard-boiled eggs to your liking.

Italian Beef Soup

Yields Provided: 4-6
Total Time: 30-35 minutes

Ingredients Required:

- Minced beef (1 lb.)
- Garlic clove (1)
- Beef broth (2 cups)
- Large tomatoes (2-3 or more if desired)
- Carrots (1 cup)
- Spinach (2 cups)
- Salt & black pepper (.25 tsp. each)

Preparation Technique:

1. Prep the veggies. Mince the garlic and beef, rinse and tear the spinach, and cube the zucchini. Slice the carrots.
2. Toss and brown the beef in a stockpot using the medium-high temperature setting. Pour in the broth, tomatoes, carrots, pepper, and salt.
3. Lower the heat, place a lid on the pot, and simmer for about 15 minutes.
4. Stir in the zucchini and cover to cook the soup until it's tender.
5. Add the spinach to wilt for about five minutes before serving.

Jambalaya Soup

Yields Provided: 8
Total Time: 55 minutes to 1 hour

Ingredients Required:

- Bacon (4 slices)
- GF Andouille sausage/kielbasa (12 oz.)
- Garlic (2 cloves)
- Chicken breasts (2)
- Yellow onion (1 small)
- Celery (2 ribs)
- Bell pepper (1 green)
- Black pepper & salt
- Cajun seasoning (2 tsp.)
- GF flour (3 tbsp.)
- Crushed tomatoes (28 oz.)
- Water (2 cups)
- Bay leaves (2)
- GF Chicken broth (32 oz.)
- Long-grain white rice (.75 cup)
- Also Needed: Six-quart Dutch oven/Heavy-duty soup pot

Preparation Technique:

1. Chop the bacon, chicken, sausage, bell pepper, onion, and celery. Mince the garlic.
2. Add the bacon into the soup pot, setting the temperature on medium – cooking until it's crispy.
3. Put the bacon on a platter, reserving the fat, and pour in enough oil to total two tablespoons of fat in the pot.
4. Set the temperature at med-high, and add the chicken, salt, and pepper, cooking for about two minutes until it is opaque.
5. Chop and add the peppers, celery, onion, and the 88auté seasoning. Sauté it for about five minutes until they are tender. Toss in the garlic and continue to sauté them for an additional 30 seconds – or so.

6. Dust flour into the pot and simmer the soup for two minutes. Pour in the chicken broth (1-2 splashes at a time) and cook for about 15-18 minutes until it's al dente.
7. The last two to three minutes, remove the pot from the burner with the lid on to allow the rice time to finish cooking.
8. At that time, remove the top and add the bacon. Wait about ten minutes for it to thicken and serve.

Sweet Corn – Kielbasa & Potato Soup

Yields Provided: 4
Total Time: 35-45 minutes

Ingredients Required:

- Bacon (4 slices)
- Kielbasa (7 oz.)
- Carrots (.5 cup)
- Celery (1 rib)
- Shallot (1)
- Garlic (2 cloves)
- Chicken broth (2.5 cups)
- Unsweetened almond milk – 2% or higher for cow's milk (1.5 cups – divided)
- GF flour (3 tbsp.)
- Baby Yukon gold potatoes (1.5 cups)
- Fresh/frozen sweet corn (1 cup)
- Black pepper & seasoned salt (as desired)
- Green onions to garnish

Preparation Technique:

1. Prepare a six-quart dutch oven using the medium temperature setting. Cook the bacon and kielbasa until it's browned. Save the bacon grease in the pan and place the meats on a platter.
2. Thinly slice the celery and carrots. Chop the green onions, carrots, bacon, and kielbasa. Mince the garlic and dice the potatoes.
3. Toss the shallot, celery, and carrots in the pan to sauté for about eight to ten minutes. Add a small amount of broth to the pan and place the lid on top. Mix in the minced garlic to sauté for one additional minute.
4. Pour in the broth with one cup of milk. Use the med-high heat setting to heat – not boil. Fold in the potatoes and lower the temperature to medium. Simmer for five to seven minutes.

5. In the meantime, whisk the flour and ½ cup of milk until creamy.
6. Add the kielbasa and bacon into the pot and steam the soup until it's slightly thickened (5 min.).
7. Add the corn and simmer one additional minute, adding pepper and salt as desired.
8. Serve with a garnish of onions.
9. Note: Seasoned salt can be homemade also. Combine the following ingredients and place them in a shaker or jar.
    a. Salt (5 tbsp.)
    b. Onion powder (2 tsp.)
    c. Paprika (1 tbsp.)
    d. Garlic powder (2 tsp.)

CHAPTER 5: CHICKEN SPECIALTIES

Almond & Artichoke Stuffed Chicken Breasts

Yields Provided: 4
Total Time: 25 minutes

Ingredients Required:

- Artichoke hearts (1 can)
- Baby spinach (.5 cup)
- Roasted almonds (2 tbsp.)
- Parmesan (2 tbsp.)
- Orange zest (1 tsp.)
- Kosher salt and black pepper (.75 tsp. of each)
- Chicken breasts (4)
- Olive oil (2 tbsp.)

Preparation Technique:

1. Trim the chicken to remove the bones and skin. Grate the orange for zest and the parmesan. Chop the spinach and almonds.
2. Combine the zest, parmesan, almonds, artichokes, spinach, salt, and pepper.
3. Slice a two-inch pocket in each breast and stuff ¼ of the mixture into the slots. Dust each one with ½ teaspoon of pepper and salt.
4. Prepare a skillet with oil to heat over the med-high temperature setting.
5. Cook the chicken for five to seven minutes per side until it's nicely browned to your liking.
6. Serve when it's ready.

Bacon Chicken Cutlets With Sweet Potato Mash

Yields Provided: 1
Total Time: 35-40 minutes

Ingredients Required:

- Sweet potatoes (2)
- Bacon (4 strips)
- Chicken cutlets (1 lb.)
- Pepper (.25 tsp.)
- Flour (.25 cup)
- Milk (.5 cup)
- Salt (.75 tsp. divided)
- Pressed garlic (.5 tsp.)
- Low-sodium chicken broth (1 cup)
- Lemon juice (2 tbsp.)
- Steamed broccoli (3 cups)

Preparation Technique:

1. Wash the potatoes and prick them with a fork. Place in the microwave for ten minutes, turning once until it's tender.
2. Fry the bacon using the med-high temperature setting (5 min.), reserving the drippings.
3. Sprinkle the cutlets using ¼ teaspoons of the pepper and salt. Dredge them in a dish of flour.
4. Cook them using the drippings for six minutes (med-high) until it reaches an internal temperature of 165° Fahrenheit. Flip them once during the cooking cycle. Put the chicken on a platter.
5. Remove the flesh of the potato into a mixing container with ¼ teaspoon of salt and the milk. Mix it until creamy.
6. Mince and add the garlic to the skillet with the broth and juice. Simmer for about three minutes.
7. Steam the broccoli to your liking.
8. Serve the chicken with the prepared sauce, mash, bacon, and steamed broccoli as desired.

Braised Chicken Thighs With Winter Vegetables

Yields Provided: 4
Total Time: 80 minutes

Ingredients Required:

- Chicken thighs (6 or about 2.5 lb.)
- Kosher salt & freshly cracked black pepper (to your liking)
- Vegetable oil (1 tbsp.)
- Ginger (2-inch section)
- Cloves of garlic (5)
- Small shallots (8 oz.)
- Sake/dry white wine (.75 cup)
- Liquid Aminos (1 cup)
- Water (.75 cup)
- Granulated sugar (.25 cup)
  For Serving:
- Toasted sesame oil (1 tbsp.)
- Green onions
- Cooked white rice
- Toasted sesame seeds

Preparation Technique:

1. Set the oven at 425° Fahrenheit.
2. Warm the oil in a large, deep oven-proof skillet using the high-temperature setting.
3. Dust the chicken using pepper and salt. Add it to a frying pan to cook until it's deeply golden (6 min.). Transfer it to a platter.
4. Mince the ginger, garlic, and shallots and toss into the skillet. Sauté the mixture for about one minute. Pour in the wine and cook until reduced by half (3 min.). Mix in the water, soy sauce, and sugar. Let it boil.
5. Arrange the chicken in the skillet with the shallots. Transfer the skillet to the middle rack of the oven and braise the chicken (lid off) for about 35 minutes and transfer the chicken from the pan.

6. Switch the pan to the high-temperature setting and cook until the sauce is thickened or about three minutes. Pour sauce and sesame oil over chicken thighs.
7. Thinly slice the green onions. Garnish with sesame seeds and the onions. Serve with rice.

Crispy Baked Chicken Fingers

Yields Provided: 4
Total Time: 25 minutes

Ingredients Required:

- GF fine cornmeal (1 cup)
- Paprika (.5 tsp.)
- Salt (.5 tsp.)
- Eggs (2 large)
- Whole milk (.25 cup)
- Thin chicken strips (1 lb.)
- GF cornstarch (.25 cup)

Preparation Technique:

1. Warm the oven to reach 375° Fahrenheit.
2. Prepare a rimmed baking tray with a sheet of parchment baking paper.
3. Whisk the paprika in one bowl. In another, whisk the milk and eggs.
4. Place the chicken in a resealable plastic bag and dust using the cornstarch.
5. Dip the strips in the eggs and cornmeal. Arrange them on the tray to bake for six minutes. Flip them over and continue roasting for another five to nine minutes until the chicken is crispy.
6. Note: You can also place the chicken on a wire rack over a baking tray for an even crispier piece of chicken.

5 Cheese Mac & Cheese With Broccoli & Chicken

Yields Provided: 4-6
Total Time: 45-50 minutes

Ingredients Required:

- Cooked chicken (2 cups – 1-inch cubes)
- Steamed broccoli (2 cups)
- Chicken broth (2 cups)
- Butter (3 tbsp.)
- White rice flour – superfine (3-4 tbsp.)
- Heavy cream (2 cups)
- Salt (2 tsp./more as needed)
- Ground dry mustard (.25 tsp.)
- Onion flakes (3 tbsp.)
- Garlic powder (.5 tsp.)
- Black pepper (.25 tsp.)
- Grated sharp white cheddar cheese (2.5 cups)
- Other cheeses – include 1.5 cups of each:
    - Medium cheddar
    - Jarlsberg
    - Monterey Jack
- Parmesan cheese (1 cup)
- Elbow macaroni (1 lb. – GF)
- Also Needed: 3-quart casserole dish

Preparation Technique:

1. Steam the broccoli and chop it into bite-sized pieces.
2. Set the oven to warm at 350° Fahrenheit. Lightly oil the baking dish.
3. Prepare a saucepan using medium heat to melt the butter. When it's hot, pour in the flour and whisk about one minute. Also, slowly add the cream until it is thickened.
4. Continue cooking. Pour in the broth slowly until it is slightly thickened.
5. Take the pan from the burner and add the garlic powder, pepper, mustard, onion flakes, and salt. Add the parmesan and most of the other cheese (saving some for the topping).

6. Prepare a pot of boiling, salted water to cook the macaroni until it is al dente (7-8 min.). Dump it into a colander to drain and add it back to the empty pot. Add the broccoli and cheese sauce and the chicken.
7. Mix thoroughly (gently) and dump it into the casserole dish, sprinkling with the reserved cheese.
8. Bake it for about 20-25 minutes and serve.

Grilled Chicken With Warm Quinoa Salad & Carrots

Yields Provided: 4
Total Time: 35 minutes

Ingredients Required:

- Red or black quinoa (6 oz.)
- Freshly ground black pepper & salt (as desired)
- Pine nuts (.25 cup)
- Olive oil (3 tbsp.)
- Cloves of garlic (3)
- Medium red onion (half of 1)
- Medium carrots (2)
- Ground cumin (2 tsp.)
- Sherry vinegar (1 tbsp. + 1 tsp.)
- Chicken breast (2 halves)
- Small mint leaves (2 tbsp.)

Preparation Technique:

1. Remove all bones and skin from the chicken.
2. Prepare the quinoa, salt, and pepper with two cups of water in a small saucepan.
3. Place a lid on the pot and simmer using the low-temperature setting for about 15 minutes until the water is absorbed.
4. Prepare a skillet and toast the pine nuts using medium heat for about two minutes. Pour them into a plate.
5. Warm three tablespoons of oil into the pan. Sauté the garlic and onions for about five minutes. Toss in the cumin and carrots to cook for approximately five more minutes.
6. Mix in the quinoa, vinegar, salt, and pepper.
7. Drizzle the chicken with oil and thread it onto skewers, adding salt and pepper to your liking.
8. Warm the grill (high heat) and cook them for about five minutes, rotating as needed.
9. Scoop the quinoa salad onto a serving dish with a garnish of nuts and mint leaves. Add the skewered chicken and serve.

Lemon Pepper & Rosemary Rubbed Chicken

Yields Provided: 4
Total Time: 45 minutes

Ingredients Required:

- Whole coriander seeds (1 tsp.)
- Fresh rosemary (1 sprig)
- Black peppercorns (1 tsp.)
- Fresh lemon zest (2 tbsp.)
- Kosher salt (.75 tsp.)
- Butter (2 tbsp. – unsalted)
- Olive oil (1 tbsp.)
- Small chicken legs (4)
- Also Needed: Large rimmed baking sheet

Preparation Technique:

1. Warm the oven to reach 425° Fahrenheit.
2. Crush the coriander seeds and peppercorns in a small mixing container.
3. Mix in the rosemary, lemon zest, and salt. Toss and stir in the butter and oil.
4. Arrange the chicken on the baking tray. Rub it with the lemon-rosemary mixture.
5. Roast the chicken for 30 to 35 minutes. Serve as desired.

Roasted Chicken With Fennel & Lemons

Total Time: 1 hour 15 minutes
Yields Provided: 4 servings

Required Ingredients:

- Chicken (1 whole)
- Coarse salt and ground pepper (to taste)
- Lemons (2 whole)
- Fennel bulbs (2.5 whole)
- Olive oil (1 tbsp.)
- Also Needed: Large-rimmed baking tray

Preparation Technique:

1. Warm the oven to reach 400° Fahrenheit.
2. Arrange the chicken and dust with pepper and salt on the baking sheet. Stuff a lemon half in the cavity.
3. Securely tie the legs together using a piece of kitchen twine.
4. Toss in the fennel, remaining lemons, and oil onto the baking tray.
5. Roast until the juices run clear (60 to 70 min.). The chicken is done when it's internal temperature registers at 165° Fahrenheit.
6. Baste the chicken with juices from the skillet and toss in the fennel halfway through the cooking cycle.
7. Transfer the chicken to a platter and "tent" it using a sheet of aluminum foil. Wait for about ten minutes before you carve it.
8. Serve with fennel and lemons.

Spatchcocked Chicken With Tomatoes

Yields Provided: 4
Total Time: 40-45 minutes

Ingredients Required:

- Spatchcocked chicken (1 whole)
- Coarse salt and ground pepper (to your liking)
- Clove of garlic (3)
- Cherry tomatoes (1 pint)
- Dry white wine (.5 cup)
- Olive oil (1 tsp.)
- Water (.25 cup)
- Fresh basil leaves (.25 cup)

Preparation Technique:

1. Heat the oven at 500° Fahrenheit.
2. Arrange the chicken with the breast side up in a pan with garlic cloves and a shake of salt and pepper.
3. Gently pierce the cherry tomatoes and add it to the pan. Drizzle the tomatoes with the pepper, salt, and oil.
4. Pour wine and water into the pan.
5. Roast the chicken until juices run clear when pierced in the thickest parts (Internal temp at 165° Fahrenheit) about 30 minutes.
6. Wait for about five minutes before carving the bird. Sprinkle with torn – fresh basil leaves.

Tandoori Chicken Drumsticks With Cilantro-Shallot Relish

Total Time: 1 hr. 15 min.
Yields Provided: 4 servings

Required Ingredients :

- Ground cumin (1 tbsp.)
- Sweet paprika (1 tbsp.)
- Ground coriander (1 tbsp.)
- Garam masala (1 tbsp.)
- Fresh ginger (1 tbsp.)
- Turmeric (.5 tsp.)
- Garlic (4 cloves)
- Greek-style yogurt – fat-free (.25 cup)
- Lemon juice (1 tbsp.)
- Canola oil (.5 cup)
- Freshly ground pepper & kosher salt (as desired)
- Chicken (12 drumsticks)
- Coarsely chopped cilantro (.75 cup)
- Shallot (1 small)
- Distilled white vinegar (3 tbsp.)
- Also Needed: 2 large baking sheets

Preparation Technique:

1. Peel and grate the ginger and garlic.
2. Set the oven at 450° Fahrenheit. Arrange a wire rack on each of the baking trays.
3. Toast the garam masala, paprika, coriander, cumin, and turmeric in a skillet using moderately low heat, stirring; until it is fragrant (2 min.).
4. Let the spices slightly cool in a mixing container. Stir in the lemon juice, ginger, salt, pepper, garlic, yogurt, and two tablespoons of oil.
5. Slice a couple of slashes in each drumstick.
6. Toss the chicken with two tablespoons of canola oil, salt, and pepper.

7. Rub the chicken using the spiced yogurt, and arrange the chicken on the racks. Roast them for about ¾ of an hour (occasionally turning).
8. Broil the chicken six inches from the heat (5 min.) until lightly charred.
9. Stir the vinegar, shallot, cilantro, salt, and the rest of the oil (.25 cup). Serve it with the chicken.

Tangy Chicken Cacciatore – Slow Cooked

Yields Provided: 4
Total Time: 5 hours 15 minutes

Ingredients Required:

- Chicken broth (1 cup)
- Tomato paste (1 can)
- Bone-in chicken thighs (2.5 lb.)
- Red peppers (2 medium)
- Cremini (baby Bella) mushrooms (12 oz.)
- Onion (1 medium)
- Pickled cherry peppers (2)
- Garlic (2 cloves)
- Fresh rosemary (2 sprigs)
- Black pepper and salt (to your liking)
  To Finish:
- Cooked polenta
- Capers (2 tbsp.)
- Also Needed: 7-8-quart slow cooker

Preparation Technique:

1. Dust the chicken with pepper and salt. Whisk the tomato paste and broth in the slow cooker and add the chicken.
2. Fold in the rest of the fixings.
3. Securely close the lid and set the timer for five hours using the low-temperature setting. Test for doneness with an internal temperature of 165° Fahrenheit.
4. Once it's ready, add the polenta to your plate and spoon the chicken over the tops with a garnishing of capers.

Yogurt Chicken Kebabs With Tomato Salad

Yields Provided: 4
Total Time: 30 minutes

Ingredients Required:

- Plain nonfat Greek yogurt (1 cup)
- Garlic (2 cloves)
- Ground cumin (.5 tsp.)
- Kosher salt and black pepper (as needed)
- Olive oil (2 tbsp.)
- Chicken breasts (1.5 lb.)
- Tomatoes – ex. Cherry, plum, beefsteak, or grape (1 lb.)
- Shallot (1)
- Fresh flat-leaf parsley leaves (.5 cup)
- Red wine vinegar (1 tbsp.)

Preparation Technique:

1. Combine the yogurt, cumin, garlic, ½ teaspoon of salt and ¼ teaspoon of pepper in a shallow baking dish.
2. Remove the skin and bones from the chicken to thread it onto eight skewers and add them to the yogurt mixture, turning to cover. Place them in the fridge to marinate (10 min. to overnight).
3. Toss the tomatoes, shallot, parsley, vinegar, oil, and ¼ teaspoon of both the pepper and salt in a mixing container.
4. Heat a grill/grill pan using the medium-high temperature setting. Oil the grill and cook the chicken, occasionally turning, until cooked thoroughly, 8-10 minutes. Serve with the tomato salad.

CHAPTER 6: PORK FAVORITES

Apple & Onion Slow-Cooked Pulled Pork

Yields Provided: 8
Total Time: 4 hours 10 minutes

Ingredients Required:

- Pork roast (4-5 lb.)
- Apples (3 cups)
- Sweet yellow onion (1 cup)
- Garlic (2 cloves)
- Soy sauce/coconut aminos (1/3 cup)
- Optional: Pickled red onion

Preparation Technique:

1. Chop the apples and onions. Mince the garlic. Toss them into the cooker and place the pork on top.
2. Empty the sauce over it all and cook for eight to ten hours on low or four to six on the high-temperature setting.
3. Shred and serve to your liking.

Carolina BBQ Pork Chops

Yields Provided: 4
Total Time: 15-20 minutes

Ingredients Required:

The Sauce:
- Spicy brown mustard (.75 cup)
- Rice vinegar (.25 cup)
- Molasses (1 tbsp.)
- Brown sugar (3 tbsp.)
- Smoked paprika (.5 tsp.)
- Black pepper (.25 tsp.)

The Chops:
- Black pepper & salt (to your liking)

Preparation Technique:

1. Use the high-temperature setting to heat the grill.
2. Combine the fixings for the sauce, whisking thoroughly.
3. Pour about ⅓ cup of the sauce into a dish and brush it over the chops (all sides).
4. Dust them using pepper and salt to grill for three to four minutes on each side.
5. Cover with a sheet of foil and wait for five minutes before serving.

Coconut Curry Pork Meatballs

Yields Provided: 4
Total Time: 35-40 minutes

Ingredients Required:

- *The Meatballs*:
- Ground Pork (1 lb.)
- Coconut flour (2-3 tbsp.)
- Egg (1)
- Shredded carrots (.5 cup)
- Minced cilantro (.25 cup)
- Minced scallions (2)
- Grated ginger (1 tbsp.)
- Green curry paste (1 tbsp.)
- Pepper & salt (as desired)
- Coconut/avocado/sesame oil (1 tbsp.)

   The Sauce:
- Full-fat coconut milk (1 can)
- Coconut aminos (1 tbsp.)
- All-natural smooth almond butter (.5 cup)
- Fresh lime juice (1 tbsp.)
- Curry paste (1 tbsp.)
- Grated ginger (1 tsp.)
- Minced garlic (2 cloves)
   The Add-Ins – 1 of each – julienned:
- Red bell pepper
- Small carrot
   The Garnish:
- Sliced/chopped almonds
- Cilantro
- Diced green onion

Preparation Technique:

1. Combine each of the sauce fixings in a food processor until creamy.

2. Prepare the meatballs by mixing the pork, flour (2 tbsp. at a time), carrots, egg, ginger, salt, pepper, curry paste, scallions, and cilantro. Shape it into sixteen meatballs.
3. Prepare a deep skillet (med-high temp) and heat the oil.
4. Cook the meatballs until browned (5-6 min.). Set them aside.
5. Lower the setting the med-low and add the sauce. Add the meatballs to heat on low for 15 minutes.
6. Add any desired veggies after 15 minutes, and stir in the carrots and red pepper. Simmer for five minutes with the lid off.
7. Serve with a dish of zoodles or cauliflower rice with cilantro and green onions.

Crispy Oven-Fried Pork Chops

Yields Provided: 4
Total Time: 20 minutes

Ingredients Required:

The Chops:
- Pork loin chops – 1-inch thick – boneless (4)
- GF breadcrumbs plain (1 cup)
- Paprika (1 tsp.)
- GF flour (1 cup)
- Milk (.25 cup)
- Eggs – lightly beaten (3 large)
- Garlic powder (1 tsp.)
- Sea salt and black pepper (.5 tsp. of each)

The Glaze:
- Dijon mustard (1 tsp.)
- Apricot preserves (4 tbsp.)
- Cayenne pepper (.25 tsp.)
- Garlic powder (.25 tsp.)

Preparation Technique:

1. Warm the oven at 450° Fahrenheit.
2. Line a baking tray using a layer of parchment baking paper.
3. Trim the fat away from the chops.
4. Prepare three large bowls. Whisk the milk and eggs in one bowl, flour in another bowl, and breadcrumbs mixed with the spices in the last bowl.
5. Dip each pork in the egg mixture, and the flour, shaking them lightly. Dredge them through the eggs again, and lastly – the breadcrumbs.
6. Arrange each of the chops onto a sheet pan (not touching). Spray them lightly with cooking oil until the breadcrumbs are dampened.
7. Bake the chops until they reach 145° Fahrenheit (internal temp), and the breadcrumbs are browned (20-25 min.).

8. You can also whisk the fixings for the apricot glaze and use it as a dipping sauce for the chops.

Crockpot Pork Chops & Herb Gravy

Yields Provided: 4
Total Time: 5 hours 20 minutes

Ingredients Required:

- GF All-purpose flour (.25 cup)
- Dry mustard powder (1 tsp.)
- Kosher salt (.5 tsp.)
- Crushed – dried rosemary (.5 tsp.)
- Dried sage (.25 tsp.)
- Dried thyme (.5 tsp.)
- Ground black pepper (.25 tsp.)
- Boneless pork chops (4)
- Olive oil (2 tbsp.)
- Chicken broth/stock – ex. – Low-FODMAP (1.5 cups)
- GF flour (1-2 tbsp.)
- Water (1-2 tbsp.)
- Chopped parsley (as desired)

Preparation Technique:

1. Lightly spritz the inside of the pot with olive oil cooking spray.
2. Combine the pepper, sage, thyme, rosemary, salt, mustard powder, and gluten-free flour (.25 cup). Use this mixture and dip the chops.
3. Warm the oil using med-high heat in a skillet. Brown the chops for three to five minutes on each side.
4. Transfer the chops to the crockpot. Deglaze the skillet with part of the broth to remove the browned bits. Add it to the pot and close the lid.
5. Set the timer on the low-temperature setting for five hours or use the high for three hours.
6. When ready, remove the chops from the cooker.
7. Mix one tablespoon – each of water and flour. Slowly add this to the crockpot – continuously stirring. Adjust the mixture of each as needed until it's thickened.

8. Serve the delicious pork chops with a portion of gluten-free pasta.

Garlic Pot Roast

Yields Provided: 10
Total Time: Varies: 7 hours 20 minutes

Ingredients Required:

- Pork boneless loin roast (3.5 lb.)
- Vegetable oil – EVOO (1 tbsp.)
- Salt (1 tsp.)
- Pepper (.5 tsp.)
- Medium onion (1)
- Garlic (3 cloves)
- Chicken broth or water (1 cup)
- Suggested: 10-inch skillet & 3.5 to 6-quart cooker

Preparation Technique:

1. Remove all of the fat from the pork.
2. Warm the oil in a skillet using the med-high temperature setting. Add and cook the pork for about ten minutes, occasionally turning until browned on all sides.
3. Peel and mince/chop the onion & garlic in the cooker. Place pork on top and pour the broth over the pork.
4. Place the lid on the cooker. Set the timer for eight to ten hours (low heat).
5. Serve when they are tender with your favorite side dishes.

Instant Pot Ribs

Yields Provided: 4
Total Time: 33 minutes

Ingredients Required:

- Baby back ribs (1 rack)
- Chicken broth (1 cup)
- Liquid smoke (.5 tsp.)
- Garlic (4 cloves)
- Sweet onion (1)
- Dry rub – below (6 tbsp.)
- Barbecue sauce (as desired)

The Dry Rub:

- Smoked paprika (1 tsp.)
- Oregano (2 tsp.)
- Black pepper (1 tsp.)
- Onion powder (2 tsp.)
- Paprika (2 tbsp.)
- Garlic powder (2 tsp.)
- Brown sugar (2 tbsp.)

Preparation Technique:

1. Rinse, remove the membrane, and pat the ribs dry.
2. Combine each of the fixings for the rub and add it to the ribs.
3. Mince the garlic and slice the onion.
4. Arrange the trivet in the Instant Pot. Measure and add the liquid smoke and broth. Arrange the ribs over the trivet with the onions and garlic.
5. Securely close the lid and set the timer for 23 minutes using the high-pressure setting. Natural-release the built-up pressure for about five minutes before opening the lid.
6. Brush them with the sauce and broil/grill the pork until charred to your liking.

Pan Ranch Pork Chops With Crispy Potatoes

Yields Provided: 4
Total Time: 40-45 minutes

Ingredients Required:

- Thick-cut bone-in pork chops (4 – 7 oz. each)
- Melted butter (2 tbsp.)
- Olive oil (3 tbsp.)
- Garlic (3 tsp.)
- Dried seasoning of ranch dressing (1-oz. pkg.)
- Halved baby red potatoes (1 lb.)

Preparation Technique:

1. Set the oven at 400° Fahrenheit.
2. Prepare a large rimmed baking tray with a layer of foil and spritz of a cooking oil spray.
3. Mince the garlic. Whisk the ranch seasoning, garlic, butter, and oil.
4. Slice the potatoes into halves and arrange in a single layer on the baking tin. Drizzle with half of the oil mixture.
5. Toss and bake them for 15 minutes. Transfer the potatoes from the oven and add the chops. Brush the pork with the remainder of the oil mix. Bake them for another 10-15 minutes. If you like it crispier, place it under the broiler (2-3 min.).

Parmesan-Crusted Oven-Baked Pork Chops

Yields Provided: 4
Total Time: 25 minutes

Ingredients Required:

- Pork chops – boneless (4 @ ½ to 1-inch thick)
- Shredded parmesan cheese (.5 cup)
- GF Breadcrumbs (.5 cup)
- Italian seasoning (1 tsp.)
- Garlic powder (.5 tsp.)
- Pepper (.25 tsp.)
- Salt (.5 tsp.)
- Olive oil (as needed)

Preparation Technique:

1. Set the oven temperature at 400° Fahrenheit.
2. Use a large shallow container to prepare the pepper, salt, garlic powder, cheese, and breadcrumbs.
3. Dab the chops dry with a paper towel.
4. Spritz the chops with an olive oil spray and dip them in the breadcrumbs, pressing it fully to cover.
5. Pour several tablespoons of oil into a cast-iron skillet using the high-temperature setting. Brown the pork three to four minutes per side.
6. Arrange the skillet in the oven. Bake it for 15 to 20 minutes and serve.

Pork Or Lamb Pilaf With Raisins & Apricots

Yields Provided: 4
Total Time: 1 hour 10-15 minutes

Ingredients Required:

- Margarine/butter (2 tbsp.)
- Long/short-grain rice (1 cup)
- Yellow onion (1 large)
- Fresh ginger (2 tbsp.)
- Garlic (2 cloves)
- GF Vegetable/beef stock (2 cups)
- Olive/vegetable oil (3 tbsp.)
- Pork loin/Boneless leg of lamb (1 lb. into ¾-inch cubes)
- Black pepper (1/8 tsp.)
- Salt (.25 tsp.)
- Zucchini (2 small)
- Dried apricots (.5 cup)
- Small halved mushrooms (4 oz.)
- Golden/dark raisins (.5 cup)
- Minced parsley (.5 cup)

Preparation Technique:

1. Mince the ginger and garlic. Chop the apricot and zucchini.
2. Prepare a saucepan and melt the butter. Add the onion, rice, one tablespoon of ginger, and garlic. Sauté them for about three to four minutes.
3. Pour in the stock and wait for it to boil. Set the temperature on low and cover the pot. Simmer for about half an hour until most of the liquid has been absorbed.
4. In a 12-inch skillet, warm one tablespoon of oil (high temp) for about a minute. Dust the meat with pepper and salt, adding it to the skillet to brown on each side (10 min.).
5. Drain the meat on a towel-lined platter.
6. Meanwhile, add the rest of the ginger and zucchini into the skillet and sauté it for about three minutes. Toss in the mushrooms to sauté about three to four minutes. Set them aside.

7. Combine the raisins and apricots with the rice and cover. Continue cooking until the liquid is absorbed (10 min.). Fold in the meat and mix everything together. Toss well and heat using the medium temperature setting (lid off).
8. Serve with the minced parsley.

Pork Tenderloin With Onions & Peppers

Yields Provided: 3-4
Total Time: 25-30 minutes

Ingredients Required:

- Coconut oil (1 tbsp.)
- Caraway seeds (1 tbsp.)
- Pork loin (1 lb.)
- Black pepper (.25 tsp.)
- Sea salt (.5 tsp.)
- Red onion (1)
- Red bell peppers (2)
- Garlic cloves (4)
- Chicken broth (1/4 to 1/3 cup)

Preparation Technique:

1. Rinse the veggies. Thinly slice the onion and peppers. Mince the garlic.
2. Slice the pork and dust with salt, pepper, and seeds.
3. Warm a skillet using the medium temperature setting.
4. Pour in the oil and add the pork to slightly brown. Toss in the mushrooms and onions and sauté until they are translucent.
5. Add the garlic, peppers, and broth. Simmer until they are thoroughly cooked.

Smothered Pork Chops

Yields Provided: 4
Total Time: 35 minutes

Ingredients Required:

- Regular long-grain rice (1 cup – uncooked – white)
- Olive oil (1 tbsp.)
- Bone-in pork loin chops ¾-inch thick (6/about 2 lb.)
- Ground black pepper and salt (.5 tsp. of each)
- Garlic (2 cloves)
- French onion soup – ex. Progresso Vegetable Classics (18.5 oz. can)
- Cornstarch (2 tbsp.)

Preparation Technique:

1. Finely chop the garlic.
2. Cook the rice before you begin.
3. Warm a skillet to heat the oil using the med-high temperature setting.
4. Sauté the garlic, salt, and pepper with the chops for four to five minutes per side.
5. Whisk the soup and cornstarch and pour it over the pork. Wait for it to get hot and lower the setting to medium.
6. Place a lid on the pan and cook it for 10-15 minutes (160° Fahrenheit internally) and serve.

CHAPTER 7: SEAFOOD SPECIALTIES

Chettinad Crab Masala

Yields Provided: 3
Total Time: 25 minutes

Ingredients Required:

To Roast & Grind:
- Oil (1 tbsp.)
- Fennel seeds (1 tbsp.)
- Peppercorns (2 tbsp.)
- Cumin seeds (1 tsp.)
- Coriander seeds (1 tbsp.)
- Dry red chilies (6)
- Onion (1)
- Tomatoes (2)

The Curry:
- Oil (1 tbsp.)
- Ginger-garlic paste (1 tbsp.)
- Curry leaf (1)
- Crab (.5 kg/1.1 lb.)
- Spring curry leaf (1)
- Fennel seeds (1 tsp.)

To Garnish:
- Coriander leaves (1 tsp.)

Preparation Technique:

1. Pour the oil, cumin seeds, peppercorns, coriander seeds, fennel seeds, into a skillet, and sauté them for a minute.
2. Toss in the dry red chilies to sauté for a second or two.
3. Mince and toss in the onions to sauté until they're translucent. Pour in the chopped tomato and sauté it until the tomato is mushy.

4. Wait for the mix to cool and mash it into a fine paste, adding about ¼ of a cup of water. Set it aside for now.
5. Warm the oil and toss in the seasonings, curry leaves, and fennel. Add the garlic-ginger paste (recipe below).
6. Sauté the mixture for two to three minutes and mix in the ground onion tomato masala.
7. Stir it for five to six minutes. (Add water as needed to prevent sticking.)
8. Adjust seasonings as desired and add the pieces of crab – immersing it in the masala.
9. Put a top on the pot and simmer the crab for eight to ten minutes – intermittently stirring.
10. Extinguish the heat when the color of the masala is slightly darker.
11. Sprinkle a few of the chopped coriander leaves over it and serve.

Ginger Garlic Paste

Yields Provided: 16
Total Time: 10 minutes

Ingredients Required:

- Garlic (4 oz.)
- Fresh ginger root (4 oz.)
- Olive oil (1 tbsp./as needed)

Preparation Technique:

1. Measure, rinse, and toss the ginger and garlic into a food processor.
2. Pulse it to blend, adding oil as needed for a smooth paste.
3. Use it now or place it in the fridge or freeze it for later.

Coconut Shrimp

Yields Provided: 4
Total Time: 1 hr. 35 min.

Required Ingredients:

- Jumbo shrimp (1 lb.)
- GF all-purpose flour (1 cup)
- Unsweetened full-fat coconut milk (13 – 1/3 oz. can)
- Sweetened coconut shreds (8 oz.)

Preparation Technique:

1. Rinse, peel, and remove the veins from the shrimp. Leave the tails on jumbo shrimp.
2. Measure and add the coconut milk, flour, and coconut shreds into three individual containers.
3. Whisk the coconut milk until it's thoroughly blended.
4. Dredge the shrimp through the flour and shake off any excess flour.
5. Dip them in the milk and toss them with the coconut and put them on a platter.
6. Repeat the process with all of the remaining shrimp, and then place the plate in the fridge to chill for one to two hours.
7. Pour the oil into a deep skillet. Add and cook the shrimp until browned for three to five minutes. Flip them over about halfway through and continue cooking another two to three minutes.
8. Transfer the shrimp to a paper towel-lined plate to drain slightly before serving.

Fish Fry With Shallots & Coconut

Yields Provided: 2
Total Time: 55 minutes

Ingredients Required:

- Fish (5 slices)
- Coconut oil (2 tbsp.)
- Salt (as desired)
- Marinade # 1
  - Chilli powder (2 tbsp.)
  - Turmeric powder (.5 tsp.)
  - Lemon/ tamarind juice (2 tsp.)
- Marinade #2
  - Coconut (3 tbsp.)
  - Shallots (6 to 7)
  - Fennel seeds (1 to 2 tbsp.)

Preparation Technique:

1. Thoroughly clean and rinse the fish. Marinate them in the salt, juice, turmeric, and chili powder for about 30 minutes.
2. Grind the fennel, coconut, and shallots into a coarse mixture and cover the fish.
3. Marinate for an additional half-hour.
4. Warm the oil in a skillet and fry the fish for five minutes per side and serve.

Flounder With Orange Coconut Oil

Yields Provided: 6
Total Time: 20-25 minutes

Ingredients Required:

- Flounder (3.5 lb.)
- White wine (3 tbsp.)
- Lemon juice (3 tbsp.)
- Coconut oil (3 tbsp.)
- Black pepper (1 tsp.)
- Parsley (3 tbsp.)
- Salt (.5 tsp.)
- Chopped scallions (.5 cup)
- Orange zest (2 tbsp.)

Preparation Technique:

1. Warm the oven to reach 325° Fahrenheit.
2. Dust the fish using pepper and salt. Place it in a baking dish with a sprinkle of orange zest.
3. Melt the coconut oil and mix in the scallions and parsley. Dump it over the fish and add the wine.
4. Bake for 15 minutes and serve with a bit of juice on the side.

GF Crab Cakes

Yields Provided: 9/18 small cakes
Total Time: 25-30 minutes

Ingredients Required:

- Large cloves garlic (2 to 3)
- Sweet yellow onion (1 small)
- Olive oil (2 tbsp.)
- Gluten-free crackers (15)
- Egg (1 large)
- Old Bay seasoning (1 tsp.)
- Mayonnaise (2 tbsp.)
- Prepared mustard (1 tbsp.)
- GF Worcestershire sauce (1 tsp.)
- GF all-purpose flour (.5 cup – for dusting crab cakes)
- Black pepper and salt (1 dash each or to taste)
- Optional: Paprika (.5 tsp.)
- Olive oil for frying (2-3 tbsp.)

Preparation Technique:

1. Mince the onion, peppers, and garlic. Sauté them in olive oil for about four minutes using the medium temperature setting. Don't brown.
2. Crush the crackers in a plastic bag using a rolling pin. Combine the crab meat, egg, crushed crackers, 129autéed vegetables, mustard, mayonnaise, Old Bay seasoning, and Worcestershire sauce. Shape it into crab cakes.
3. Combine the flour, pepper, salt, and paprika in a shallow dish. Dust each cake with flour.
4. Prepare a skillet with oil using the med-high temperature setting to brown the crabcakes.
5. Serve with your favorite side dish.

GF Lobster Cakes

Yields Provided: 4
Total Time: 20-25 minutes

Ingredients Required:

- Pre-cooked lobster (1 lb.)
- Egg (1)
- Mustard (1 tbsp.)
- Parsley (1 heaping tsp. + more if desired)
- Salt (1 dash)
- Chopped onion (.25 cup)
- Coconut flour (1.5 tbsp.)
- Almond flour/meal for coating the cakes

Preparation Technique:

1. Remove the meat from the lobster and chop the onions.
2. Whisk the egg, salt, parsley, and mustard.
3. Finely chop the lobster and onions into the egg mix.
4. Add in the coconut flour (slowly) and form it into four patties.
5. Dip each of the patties in the almond flour.
6. Prepare a skillet with a bit of oil and heat it using the low-medium temperature setting.
7. Cook until they are lightly browned and serve with your favorite side dishes.

Grilled Salmon

Yields Provided: 4
Total Time: 4 hours 15-20 minutes

Ingredients Required:

- Salmon fillets (4 – 4 oz.)
- Coconut oil (.25 cup)
- Lemon juice (2 tbsp.)
- Fish sauce (2 tbsp.)
- Green onion (2 tbsp.)
- Ginger (.75 tsp.)
- Garlic clove (1)
- Crushed red pepper flakes (.5 tsp.)
- Salt (1/8 tsp.)
- Sesame oil (.5 tsp.)

Preparation Technique:

1. Thinly slice the onion. Mince the garlic and ginger.
2. Combine all of the fixings except for the fish. Whisk them thoroughly.
3. Place the fish in a casserole dish and cover with the marinade. Marinate them for four hours.
4. Warm the grill and cook the salmon – flipping it once – until it's flaky.

Lemon-Olive Oil Pasta With Tuna

Yields Provided: 4
Total Time: 20 minutes

Ingredients Required:

- Olive oil (1 tsp. + .25 cup)
- Garlic (3 tbsp.)
- Albacore tuna (4.5 oz. can)
- Fresh pepper and salt (.25 tsp. each)
- GF cooked spaghetti
- Lemon juice (1 lemon)
- Parsley (1 bunch)

Preparation Technique:

1. Mince the garlic and drain the tuna. Roughly chop the parsley after moving the stems.
2. Warm a saucepan to heat one teaspoon of oil. Toss in the garlic to sauté for one to two minutes.
3. Stir in the pepper, salt, and tuna. Simmer for about five to seven minutes.
4. Add the cooked pasta, parsley, lemon, and rest of the oil.
5. Stir, serve and enjoy it.

Roasted Shrimp

Yields Provided: 6
Total Time: 20 minutes

Ingredients Required:

- Shrimp (2 lb.)
- Coarse salt (1 tsp.)
- Old Bay Seasoning (4 tsp.)
- Black pepper (1 tsp.)
- Juice of 1 lemon
- Olive oil (1 tbsp.)

Preparation Technique:

1. Set the oven at 400° Fahrenheit.
2. Peel, clean, and devein the shrimp (tails on them).
3. Toss the shrimp in a pan with each of the fixings.
4. Roast them for about five to six minutes. Serve.

Seafood Crepes

Yields Provided: 4
Total Time: 50 minutes

Ingredients Required:

Gluten-Free Crepes:
- Non-dairy milk (.5 cup)
- Egg (1)
- Tapioca flour (.25 cup)
- Brown rice flour (.25 cup)
- Avocado oil (1.5 tsp.)
- Sea salt (1/8 tsp.)
-

Filling:
- Asparagus frozen (8 spears)
- Avocado oil (1 tbsp.)
- Butter (1 tbsp.)
- Clove of garlic (1)
- Raw shrimp, or seafood of choice (3/4 pound – 400g)
- Crimini mushrooms (4 sliced)
- Nutmeg (1 pinch)
- Black pepper & sea salt (a pinch)
- Lemon juice (1 tbsp.)

Hollandaise Sauce:
- Egg yolks (3)
- Lemon juice (1 tbsp.)
- Hot water (1 tbsp.)
- Butter (.5 lb./227g)
- Cayenne pepper and sea salt (1 pinch of each)

Preparation Technique:

1. Mix the crepe fixings in a blender until smooth.
2. Prepare the crepes in a skillet using the medium temperature setting.
3. Make the filling. Cook asparagus and set it aside to stay warm.

4. Warm the butter and oil in a skillet using the med-high temperature setting. Mince and add the garlic.
5. Slice and add the mushrooms, stirring. Add shrimp and stir until they turn pink.
6. Transfer the pan to the countertop and mix in the salt, pepper, nutmeg, and lemon juice.
7. Prepare the sauce by combining the egg yolks, lemon juice, and hot water to a tall, narrow container. Warm the butter just until it starts to bubble. Pour it into a heatproof pouring cup.
8. Using a blender, combine the lemon juice, egg yolks, and hot water. While the mixer is running, add in the melted butter, salt, and cayenne pepper.
9. Dump the sauce into a saucepan to keep it warm so it will thicken.
10. Make crepes and prepare the filling. Keep them warm.
11. Prepare the hollandaise sauce. Place two asparagus spears across the center of each of four crepes. Spoon the filling over them and drizzle a little hollandaise sauce over the filling. Fold each side in over the filling.
12. Serve two crepes on each serving plate with a drizzle of warm hollandaise sauce.

Seared Chilean Sea Bass

Yields Provided: 4
Total Time: 30 minutes

Ingredients Required:

- Chilean sea bass fillets (1 lb.)
- Fish sauce (.5 – 1 tsp.)
- Lemon juice (1 splash)
- Pepper & Salt (as desired)
- Avocado oil (1 tsp.)
-
  The Sauce:
- Sesame oil (1 tsp.)
- Minced ginger (1 tbsp.)
- Rice vinegar (2 tbsp.)
- Maple syrup (.5 tbsp.)
- Fish sauce (2 tbsp.)
- Olive oil (1 tbsp.)
- Lime juice (2 tbsp.)
- Thai chili garlic sauce/Sriracha (1-2 tbsp.)
  The Spinach:
- Sesame oil (1 tsp.)
- Spinach (10 oz.)
- Sesame seeds (1-2 tsp.)

Preparation Technique:

1. Rinse and pat dry the sea bass fillets. Cut them into four ¾-inch thick pieces. Drizzle them using the fish sauce, lemon juice, salt, and pepper as desired.
2. Warm a cast-iron skillet using the high-temperature setting until it's almost smoking. Lower the temp to med-high and add one teaspoon avocado oil.
3. When it's hot, add the bass fillets in a single layer to cook for four to six minutes per side (without moving them) until browned.

4. Whisk the sauce fixings (fish sauce, lime juice, minced ginger, rice vinegar, agave, one teaspoon sesame oil, olive oil, and sambal oelek) until smooth.
5. Remove the cooked fish and set it aside.
6. Use the same pan for cooking the spinach in one teaspoon of sesame oil until just wilted (1 min.).
7. Divide spinach onto four plates, sprinkle with sesame seeds, top with the bass, and drizzle with sauce.

Shrimp – Asparagus & Quinoa Stir Fry

Yields Provided: 4
Total Time: 15-20 minutes

Ingredients Required:

- Olive oil (1 tbsp.)
- Garlic (1 tbsp.)
- Cornstarch (1 tsp.)
- Lemon (zest – 1 tsp. + juice – 3 tbsp.)
- Asparagus (12 oz.)
- Shrimp: Fresh or thawed frozen medium-jumbo (12 oz.)
- Dry white wine (.25 cup)
- Cooked – chilled quinoa (2 cups)

Preparation Technique:

1. Finely grate and remove the juice from the lemon.
2. Mince the garlic and whisk with the lemon juice, zest, cornstarch, and oil. Toss it into a skillet and sauté using the med-high temperature setting until it is bubbly.
3. Trim the asparagus to one-inch pieces, and add it to the skillet to cook until slightly softened (2 min.).
4. Peel, devein, and add the shrimp into the mixture with the wine. Cook them until they are opaque (2-3 min.).
5. Mix in the quinoa to simmer for two to three minutes until it's heated and serve.
6. Note: Prepare the quinoa a day in advance and chill it in the fridge until the time to prepare the dish. You can also use long-grain rice if desired.

CHAPTER 8: BEEF FAVORITES

Beef & Bean Casserole

Yields Provided: 6
Total Time: 50 minutes

Ingredients Required:

- Ground Beef (1 lb.)
- Chopped onion (.5 cup)
- Mushroom/chicken soup (1 cup)
- Salt (1 tsp.)
- Garlic powder (1/8 tsp.)
- Frozen green beans (16 oz.)
- Shredded cheddar cheese (as desired)
- GF tater tots (8 oz.)

Preparation Technique:

1. Warm the oven to reach 350° Fahrenheit.
2. Cook and drain the beans.
3. Prepare the onion and beef in a skillet and drain the fat.
4. Add the soup in a saucepan with the garlic and salt. Mix and add the onions and beef.
5. Dump it into a two-quart dish, adding half of the beans in the bottom with a layer of meat, cheese, beans, and beef. Top it off with the tater tots.
6. Bake the casserole for about 30 minutes and serve.
7. Enjoy it for lunch or dinner. You can also use veggie crumbles instead of the meat for a change of pace!

Beef & Broccoli Stir Fry

Yields Provided: 6
Total Time: 50 minutes

Ingredients Required:

The Marinade:
- Water (.25 cup)
- GF soy sauce (.25 cup)
- Garlic (2 minced)
- Ground pepper (.25 tsp.)
- Boneless round steak/stir-fry beef (1 lb.)

The Stir Fry:
- Oil (2 tbsp.)
- Broccoli florets (4 cups)
- Onion (.5 cup)
- Carrots (.5 cup)

Thee Stir Fry Sauce:
- Cold water (1 cup)
- Gluten-free soy sauce (.25 cup)
- Brown sugar (.25 cup)
- Ground ginger (1.5 tsp.)
- Sesame oil (1 tsp.)
- Optional: Red pepper flakes (.25 tsp.)
- Cornstarch (.25 cup)
- Optional: Toasted sesame seeds (1-2 tsp.)
- Optional: Sliced onion greens

Preparation Technique:

1. Do the prep. Mince the garlic. Thinly slice/chop the onion and carrots. Slice the steak into 3-inch strips.
2. Make the marinade. Whisk the water, soy sauce, garlic, and black pepper. Add the stir-fry beef strips and marinate for at least half an hour.
3. Stir Fry: In a large frying pan or wok, heat two tablespoons of oil over med-high heat. Fold in the beef and marinade, and fry until the meat is no longer pink (3-5 min.).

4. Add the onions and carrots, and fry, while continuing to stir for another two minutes.
5. Add the broccoli and continue stirring and frying for one more minute.
6. In a glass measuring cup, whisk the cup cold water, soy sauce, brown sugar, ginger, sesame oil, red pepper flakes, and cornstarch. Pour this mixture over the beef & broccoli mixture, and cook until sauce thickens (2-3 min.).
7. Serve immediately over hot rice. Sprinkle with toasted sesame seeds and onion greens before serving.

Beef Stroganoff

Yields Provided: 4
Total Time: 55-60 minutes

Ingredients Required:

- Rice flour (2 tbsp.)
- Black pepper (as desired)
- Fresh marjoram leaves – divided (2 tsp.)
- Round tip steak (.75 lb.)
- Butter (2 tbsp.)
- Yellow onion (1 large)
- Baby Bella or white mushrooms (8 oz.)
- Garlic cloves (2)
- Beef broth, divided (1.25 cups)
- Tomato sauce (3 tbsp.)
- Sour cream (.5 cup)
- Hot cooked brown rice (2.5 cups)

Preparation Technique:

1. Trim the beef and cut it into 1.5-inch pieces. Cut the onion in half and slice it. Mince the garlic and quarter the mushrooms.
2. In a large resealable plastic bag, combine the rice flour, one teaspoon of the marjoram, and pepper. Add the beef, seal the bag, and turn to coat; set it aside for now.
3. In a large nonstick skillet, melt the butter over med-high heat.
4. Remove the beef from the flour mixture, reserving the flour mixture. Working in batches if needed, add the meat to the skillet. Cook and stir it until evenly browned (2-3 min.).
5. Push the beef to the edge of the skillet, and reduce the heat to medium. Add in the onion, mushrooms, and garlic. Cook and stir it for three minutes.
6. Stir in ¾ cup of the broth and remaining one teaspoon marjoram. Reduce the heat; simmer, covered, 35–40 minutes or until beef is tender.

7. Stir reserved flour mixture into remaining ½ cup broth in a mixing bowl. Stir the broth mixture and tomato sauce in a skillet, cooking over medium heat until thickened.
8. Stir in sour cream, and cook just until heated. Serve over rice while it's still piping hot.

Beef Taco Bowls

Yields Provided: 4
Total Time: 30 minutes

Ingredients Required:

- Lean ground beef (1 lb.)
- Small onion (half of 1) or Shallot (1)
- Black pepper and salt (as desired)
- Coleslaw mix (12 oz.)
- Taco seasoning (1 recipe – see below)
- Chicken/beef broth or water (.25 cup)

Toppings Suggested:
- Salsa
- Guacamole
- Sour Cream
- Tortilla chips
- Green onions
- Shredded cheese

Preparation Technique:

1. Prep a large skillet using the med-high temperature setting. Add the beef, salt, pepper and shallot/onion; brown and drain the fat.
2. Add it back to the skillet and mix in the coleslaw mix. Sauté until it's tender (3-4 min.).
3. Stir in the taco seasoning, water/broth, and stir to combine.
4. Serve as desired.

Taco Seasoning – For One Pound of Beef

Yields Provided: One recipe
Total Time: 5 minutes

Ingredients Required:

- Chili powder (2.5 tsp.)
- Cumin (.75 tsp.)
- Dried oregano (1/8 tsp.)
- Regular/smoked paprika (.25 tsp.)
- Garlic & Onion powder (1/8 tsp. of each)
- Red chili pepper flakes (1/8 tsp.)
- Black pepper and salt (.25 tsp. each)

Preparation Technique:

1. Whisk each of the seasonings in a mixing container.
2. Store in a closed container until it's time to use it.

Cheeseburger Casserole

Yields Provided: 6-8
Total Time: 45 minutes

Ingredients Required:

- Ground beef (2 lb.)
- Large onion (1)
- Shredded cheddar cheese (1 cup)
- Mayonnaise (.25 cup)
- Ketchup (.5 cup)
- Mustard (2 tbsp.)
- GF tater tots - frozen (2 lb.)
- Also Needed: 9x13 baking dish

Preparation Technique:

1. Set the oven to reach 375° Fahrenheit.
2. Chop the onion and shred the cheese.
3. Prepare a skillet to cook the onion and beef. Combine all of the fixings (omit the tater tots).
4. Dump the mixture into the dish and add a layer of tater tots.
5. Bake it for about half an hour.

Crunchy Taco Hamburger Helper

Yields Provided: 5
Total Time: 30-35 minutes

Ingredients Required:

- Lean ground beef (1 lb.)
- Large shallot (1) or Small chopped onion (half of one)
- Taco seasoning packet (1 - don't add water)
- Salsa (.5 cup)
- Chicken broth (1.75 cups)
- Long-grain white rice - ex. jasmine/basmati (1 cup)
- Shredded sharp cheddar cheese (1 cup)

Suggested Toppings:
- Additional salsa
- Crushed tortilla chips
- Chopped green onions
- Side of sliced avocado

Preparation Technique:

1. Prepare a skillet using the med-high temperature setting. Brown the onion and beef. Mix in the salsa, seasoning, and chicken broth.
2. Wait for it to boil. Stir in the rice and place a lid on the pot. Reduce the heat setting to low.
3. Cook slowly until the rice is tender (15-20 min.). Remove it from the burner and fold in the cheese until it's melted.
4. Place the top back on the pot and wait for five minutes before serving.

Mexican Quinoa & Beef - Slow-Cooked

Yields Provided: Varies 4-6
Total Time: Varies - 4 hours

Ingredients Required:

- Ground beef/turkey (2 lb.)
- Yellow onion (1 medium)
- Bell pepper (1 yellow)
- Garlic (2 cloves)
- Red quinoa (1 cup)
- Black beans (15 oz. can)
- Diced tomatoes with juice (14.5 oz. can)
- Homemade taco seasoning (2 tbsp.)
- Water (2 cups)
- Lime juice (1 tbsp.)

  Optional Toppings:
- Sliced green onions
- Sour cream

Preparation Technique:

1. Chop the peppers and onion. Mince the garlic and prepare the taco seasoning. Rinse and drain the black beans.
2. Sauté the beef with the bell pepper and onions until softened. Stir in the garlic to sauté for one additional minute.
3. Toss all of the fixings, except for the juice, in a lightly greased cooker.
4. Stir and securely close the lid and set the timer for three to four hours on the high setting. Check it after about two hours to see if it needs more liquids.
5. Serve with the lime juice and other toppings to your liking.

Mini Philly Cheesesteak Meatloaves

Yields Provided: 4
Total Time: 35-40 minutes

Ingredients Required:

- Butter (1.5 tbsp.)
- Olive oil (1.5 tbsp.)
- Yellow onion (1 small)
- Green pepper (1 small)
- Garlic (2 cloves)
- Black pepper and salt
- Egg (1 whisked)
- Gluten-free Worcestershire sauce - ex. Lea & Perrins (1 tbsp.)
- Lean ground beef (1 lb.)
- Crushed Rice Chex (.5 cup)
- Provolone cheese (3 oz./Cut into ¼-inch cubes)

Preparation Technique:

1. Set the oven to warm at 425° Fahrenheit. Cover a baking tray using a layer of foil and a spritz of cooking oil spray.
2. Warm the butter and oil in a skillet using the med-high temperature setting. Mince and sauté the onions and salt until golden (3-4 min.).
3. Dice and add the peppers to sauté (3-4 min.). Lower the heat and mince and add the garlic to sauté for about 30 more seconds. Dump the veggies in a platter to slightly cool.
4. Mix the egg, beef, Rice Chex, salt, pepper, Worcestershire sauce, peppers, and onions.
5. Divide into four portions to form loaves and place them in the prepared pan.
6. Bake it for about 20-22 minutes and serve with your favorite sides.

Pepper Steak - Slow Cooker

Yields Provided: 4-6
Total Time: Varies (3-4 hours)

Ingredients Required:

- Coconut oil (3 tbsp.)
- Beef broth (1 cup)
- Beef sirloin (2 lb.)
- Minced garlic (1 tbsp.)
- Tapioca flour (1 tbsp.)
- Carrots (2 cups)
- Chopped onions (.5 cup)
- Chopped tomatoes (1 cup)
- Salt (1 tsp.)

Preparation Technique:

1. Chop the tomatoes and onions.
2. Mince the garlic and cook it in a skillet with the oil.
3. Cut the sirloin into two-inch strips and brown with the garlic.
4. Add everything to the slow cooker and cover.
5. Cook for six to eight hours on low or use high for three to four hours.
6. Serve as desired when it's ready!

CHAPTER 9: SNACKS & TASTY APPETIZERS

Bacon-Wrapped Figs

Yields Provided: 6
Total Time: 20 minutes

Ingredients Required:

- Figs (12)
- Thin-cut bacon/pancetta (3-6 pieces)

Preparation Technique:

1. Rinse and pat dry the figs. Remove any stems.
2. Slice the bacon in half.
3. Wrap each fig with a strip of bacon.
4. Heat a large skillet using the med-high temperature setting.
5. Cook them until each side is browned and crispy as desired.
6. Place them on several layers of paper towels to drain the fat oils before serving them.

Bacon-Wrapped Jalapeno Poppers

Yields Provided: 4
Total Time: 35-40 minutes

Ingredients Required:

- Jalapenos (12)
- Bacon (1 lb.)
- Cream/goat cheese (8 oz.)
- Balsamic glaze/ barbecue sauce (.25 cup)
- Garlic salt (as desired)

Preparation Technique:

1. Set the oven at 425° Fahrenheit. Slice the jalapenos in half - lengthwise- and discard the pith and seeds. It's recommended to wear gloves during the process.
2. Place the prepared jalapenos on a baking tray and fill them with cheese using a piping bag.
3. Sprinkle them with the salt and wrap with ½ slice of bacon.
4. Baste the tops with the sauce.
5. Set a timer to bake them for 20 minutes until it's crispy to your liking.

Buffalo Quinoa Bites

Yields Provided: 30-32 bites
Total Time: 50-55 minutes

Ingredients Required:

- Cooked quinoa (2 cups)
- Eggs (4)
- Tomato paste (3 tbsp.)
- Sea salt - fine grain (1 tsp.)
- Garlic powder (.5 tsp.)
- Ground black pepper (.25 tsp.)
- Cayenne pepper (.5 tsp.)
- Paprika (.5 tsp.)
- Breadcrumbs - ex. - Gillian's GF (1 cup)
- Mozzarella (30 - ½-inch cubes)

The Sauce:
- Butter (½ stick or 4 oz.)
- Hot sauce - ex. Frank's Red Hot (.5 cup)

Preparation Technique:

1. Warm the oven at 350°Fahrenheit. Cover a baking tray using a layer of parchment baking paper.
2. Combine/whisk the eggs, tomato paste, quinoa, garlic powder, salt, black pepper, and paprika into a mixing container.
3. Mix in the breadcrumbs and wait two to three minutes.
4. Scoop one heaping tablespoon of the quinoa mixture to make the quinoa balls. Push a cube of mozzarella into the middle of the ball and close it. Repeat the process until the mixture is gone, placing them on the prepared tray.
5. Set the timer to bake for 15 minutes. Mix the hot sauce and butter in a saucepan using the medium-temperature setting.
6. Remove the baking tray from the oven and top with buffalo sauce.
7. Bake them for another eight minutes.
8. Serve with celery sticks and blue cheese dip as desired.

Cheesy Mashed Potato Balls

Yields Provided: 2-3
Total Time: 30-45 minutes

Ingredients Required:

- Mashed potato (2 boiled)
- Spring onions (2 tbsp.)
- Coriander leaves (2 tbsp.)
- Ginger (2 tsp.)
- Garlic (2 tsp.)
- Green chili (1)
- Coriander powder (1 tsp.)
- Chilli powder (2 tsp.)
- Garam masala (1 tsp.)
- Pepper (2 tsp.)
- Cumin powder (1 tsp.)
- Cheese (.5 cup)
- Salt (as desired)
  The Batter:
- Maida (.5 cup)
- Chilli powder (1 tsp.)
- Rice flour (2 tbsp.)
- Pepper (.5 tsp.)
- Water (1 cup)

Preparation Technique:

1. Boil and peel the potatoes. Finely chop the green chili.
2. Combine the cheese fixings with the potatoes and form them into balls. Leave them on a tray for now.
3. Prepare the batter by combining the seasonings, flour, and maida in a mixing container. Add water a little at a time, whisking to prevent it from being lumpy.
4. Warm the oil in a wok.
5. Dip the potato balls into the batter - one at a time - to fry them using the medium temperature setting.
6. Remove them and drain on paper towels to serve.

Espinacas a la Catalana

Yields Provided: 4
Total Time: 6-8 minutes

Ingredients Required:

- Spinach (2 cups)
- Cashews (3 tbsp.)
- Garlic cloves (2)
- Dried currants (3 tbsp.)
- Avocado or olive oil (as needed)

Preparation Technique:

1. Peel and mince the garlic. Add a bit of oil into a skillet to heat (medium temp). Toss in the garlic to sauté for about one to two minutes.
2. Rinse and snip the stems from the spinach and steam it for a few minutes.
3. Fold in the currants and cashews to sauté for about one minute. Fold in the spinach. Toss it thoroughly with the oil and salt before serving.

Macho Nachos

Yields Provided: 8
Total Time: 50-55 minutes

Ingredients Required:

- Lean ground beef (1 lb.)
- GF corn tortilla chips (12 oz.)
- GF taco seasoning (2 tbsp.)
- Grated Monterey Jack/Cheddar cheese (12 oz.)
- Red/orange Bell pepper (.5 cup - chopped)
- Sweet yellow onion (.5 cup - chopped)
- Sliced black olives (.5 cup - blot dry)
- Pickled Jalapeno peppers (.5 cup - blot dry)
- Green onions (.5 cup - thinly sliced)
- Roma tomatoes (.5 cup - chopped and blot dry)
- Fresh cilantro (.25 cup)
- Also Needed: 13 x 9-inch baking dish

Preparation Technique:

1. Brown the beef in a cast-iron skillet. Drain the fat and stir in the taco seasoning. Set it aside for now.
2. Set the oven at 400° Fahrenheit.
3. Spread a layer of one-third of the corn chips in the baking dish.
4. Add one-third of the cooked hamburger evenly over the chips.
5. Lastly, sprinkle one-third of each (chopped jalapenos, yellow onions, bell pepper, green onions, black olives, and tomatoes) over the hamburger.
6. Sprinkle one-third of a cup of shredded cheese over the vegetables.
7. Continue with two more layers.
8. Bake them until the cheese melts (20 min.).
9. Serve with a sprinkle freshly chopped cilantro.

Spinach Balls

Yields Provided: 40 balls
Total Time: 20-25 minutes

Ingredients Required:

- Frozen chopped spinach (16 oz.)
- Butter (6 tbsp.)
- Eggs (3)
- Cheddar cheese (.75 cup - grated)
- Parmesan cheese (3 oz. - finely grated)
- Sweet paprika (.5 tsp.)
- Dry Italian spice mix (.5 tsp.)
- Fresh parsley (1/3 cup)
- Corn Chex cereal (4 cups/ finely crushed - 1.5 cups)
- GF flour (3 tbsp.)

Preparation Technique:

1. Set the oven temperature at 350° Fahrenheit. Cover two baking trays with a layer of parchment baking paper.
2. Thaw, chop the spinach and place it into a colander. Use a wooden spoon to press the spinach and remove as much moisture as possible. Twist it dry in a bunch of paper towels or a tea towel.
3. Melt and add the butter and eggs in a bowl to beat until the mixture frothy. Add in the cheeses, spices, and minced parsley, and spinach. Mix well. Stir the flour and cereal, stirring until the clumps of spinach are removed.
4. Scoop the mixture, rolling it in your hands to make the balls. Put them onto the prepared baking trays and set the timer to bake for 15 minutes.
5. Note: Measure the four cups of cereal and crush it to reach 1.5 cups of breadcrumbs.

Spinach & Artichoke Risotto Balls

Yields Provided: 10
Total Time: 70 minutes (chilling time not counted)

Ingredients Required:

- GF Chicken broth (4 cups)
- Olive oil (2 tbsp.)
- Shallots (2 small or 1/3 cup)
- Garlic (2 cloves)
- Fine sea salt
- Arborio rice (1.5 cups)
- Dry white wine (.5 cup)
- Parmesan cheese - freshly grated (.5 cup)
- Artichoke hearts in olive oil (9.87 oz. jar)
- Fresh baby spinach (2 cups)
- GF flour (1 cup)
- Pepper & salt (to your liking)
- Eggs (2)
- Water (2 tsp.)
- GF Italian breadcrumbs (2 cups)
- Canola oil (as needed for frying)

  For Serving:
- Marinara sauce
- Shaved parmesan cheese

Preparation Technique:

1. Chop the shallots and mince the garlic. Drain and chop the artichoke hearts.
2. Heat the chicken broth in a saucepan.
3. Warm the olive oil in a large sauté pan using the medium temperature setting. Once the pan is hot, toss in the shallots, garlic, pepper, and salt to sauté about three minutes.
4. Pour in the rice to sauté an additional two to three minutes until the rice is toasted.
5. Pour and stir the wine until it's almost evaporated.

6. Pour in the broth (.5 cup at a time). After the rice absorbs it, add another half cup. Stir and let it finish cooking until it's firm or as desired (al dente).
7. Fold in the spinach, artichokes, and grated parmesan. Dump the risotto into a dish and place it in the fridge overnight.
8. When it's chilled, roll it into two-inch balls (20).
9. Set up three bowls; #1 with flour, salt, and pepper; #2 - whisk the eggs and mix with water; #3 will have breadcrumbs.
10. Simply, roll each of the balls in the flour, egg, and breadcrumbs until thoroughly coated. Arrange them on a platter and continue until all are done. Pop them in the fridge for at least thirty minutes or overnight.
11. Fry Time: Warm the about three inches of oil in a large, heavy-bottom pot to reach 375° Fahrenheit).
12. Cook the risotto balls in batches until browned (2 min.). Remove and drain on paper towels. (Pop them into a 200° Fahrenheit oven to keep warm.)
13. Serve the balls hot. Garnish them using a portion of parmesan cheese and parsley. Enjoy with a warm marinara sauce for dipping.

Thai Mini Shrimp Lettuce Wraps

Yields Provided: 6/12 wraps
Total Time: 27-30 minutes

Ingredients Required:

- Baby shrimp (1 cooked - packed cup)
- Dry-roasted peanuts (1/3 cup)
- Green onions (2)
- Garlic (2 cloves)
- Ginger (2 tsp.)
- Fresh red chili (1 minced / Dried crushed chili (¼ to ½ tsp.)
- Chili powder (.5 tsp.)
- Sugar (.25 tsp.)
- Fish sauce (1 tbsp.)
- Coconut milk (3 tbsp.)
- Romaine lettuce (1 head/1 package prepared leaves)
- Fresh coriander/cilantro (1/3 cup)
- Fresh lime (half to one whole)

Preparation Technique:

1. Prepare the ingredients. Finely chop the peanuts. Mince the garlic and ginger. Slice the green onions and slice the lime into wedges.
2. Place the coconut in a dry frying pan or wok using the med-high temperature setting.
3. Dry-fry it until it is lightly browned and place it in a container to cool.
4. Be sure the shrimp are well-drained.
5. Add most of the ground peanuts to the mixing bowl, reserving one tablespoon for the topping.
6. Toss in the ginger, onions, chili, garlic, chili powder, sugar, and fish sauce. Pour in the milk and stir it again.
7. Add the toasted coconut and stir again.
8. Chop off the tops of a dozen of the romaine lettuce leaves (three to four-inch pieces) and place them on a platter.
9. Scoop an over-filled tablespoon of the shrimp mixture onto each leaf with a sprinkling of the peanuts and coconut.

Sprinkle it with fresh coriander, and serve with the wedges of lime.
10. Squeeze lime juice over the shrimp mixture and wrap them to serve.

Tuna Spring Rolls

Yields Provided: 6 rolls
Total Time: 10 minutes

Ingredients Required:

- Flaked light tuna (1 can)
- Green onions (2)
- Seasoned salt (.5 tsp.)
- Light mayonnaise (2 tbsp.)
- Leaves of lettuce
- Orange or red pepper
- Cucumber
- Spring roll wrappers

Preparation Technique:

1. Slice as many peppers and cucumber as desired.
2. Mix the tuna, mayonnaise, green onions, and seasoned salt.
3. Prepare the wrappers by running under warm water, one at a time.
4. To fill, start with a piece of the leaf lettuce to create a bed on the lower portion of the wrap.
5. Spoon on top - a row of the tuna, and lastly, place the cucumbers and peppers.
6. Fold the rolls and use a bit of water on your finger to rub the roll to make a seal. Serve as desired.

Vegan Avocado Boats

Yields Provided: 2
Total Time: 15 minutes

Ingredients Required:

- Hearts of palm (1 can)
- Green onions (.25 cup)
- Cooked quinoa (.5 cup)
- Chili pepper (1 small)
- Capers (1 tbsp.)
- Cayenne for sprinkling
- Black pepper and salt (as desired)
- Avocado (1)

    The Avocado Mayo:
    - Avocado (half of 1)
    - Coconut milk (1 tbsp.)
    - Dijon mustard (1 tsp.)
    - Minced garlic (1 small clove)
    - Olive oil (2 tbsp.)
    - Lime juice (1 tbsp.)

Preparation Technique:

1. Cut the hearts of palm into matchsticks. Dice the onions and mince the chili peppers. Slice the avocado in half and scoop out the goodies and dice into cubes.
2. Mix the mayonnaise fixings (shown above). Blend until smooth.
3. Combine the hearts of palm, quinoa, chili pepper, green onions, capers, and cubed avocado.
4. Mix in the mayo with the quinoa bowl.
5. Serve in the avocado shells.

CHAPTER 10: DELICIOUS DESSERTS

Almond Flour Cupcakes With Raspberry Frosting

Yields Provided: 6
Total Time: Varies - 1 hour 35 minutes

Ingredients Required:

- Almond flour (.25 cup)
- Coconut flour (.25 cup)
- Sea salt(.25 tsp.)
- Large eggs (3)
- Vanilla extract (1 tbsp.)
- Coconut oil (.25 cup)
- Stevia concentrated powder (.125 tsp.) or Liquid (30 drops)
- Baking soda (.25 tsp.)
- Tapioca or coconut flour (.5 tsp.)
- Chilled & canned coconut cream (13.5 oz. - 1 can)
- Liquid stevia (10 drops)
- Fresh raspberries - blended (.5 cup)

Preparation Technique:

1. Heat the oven to reach 350° Fahrenheit.
2. Use a hand or stand mixer to combine the sea salt, both types of flour, and baking soda. Whisk and toss in the eggs, stevia, coconut oil, and vanilla extract one at a time, mixing between each ingredient.
3. Arrange the cupcake liners in the pan and fill about ¾ full with batter.
4. Bake the cupcakes for 20 to 25 minutes.
5. Remove the coconut cream for the refrigerator and separate the water from the fat. Place the coconut fat into a medium mixing bowl. (Discard or save the water to drink or for another recipe.)

6. Add the tapioca /coconut flour with the stevia and the coconut cream. Beat everything until it forms stiff peaks.
7. Use a blender/food processor to crush the raspberries. Fold the fruit mixture into the frosting.
8. Cool the cupcakes for at least an hour before frosting the cupcakes using a pastry bag or spoon.

Blueberry - Coconut Flour Scones

Yields Provided: 12
Total Time: 45-50 minutes

Ingredients Required:

- Coconut flour (.5 cup)
- Almond flour (1.5 cups)
- Monk fruit sweetener (1/3 cup)
- Baking powder (1 tbsp.)
- Salt (.25 tsp.)
- Chilled butter (.25 cup)
- Blueberries - fresh or frozen (1 cup)
- *Optional*: Blackstrap molasses (.5 tsp.)
- Heavy cream (1/3 cup)
- Almond milk - unsweetened (1/3 cup)
- Eggs (2)

  Optional Glaze:
- Monk fruit sweetener (.25 cup)
- Vanilla extract (.25 tsp.)
- Lemon juice (2-3 tsp.)

Preparation Technique:

1. Mix the salt with both types of flour, sweetener, and baking powder. Cut the butter into the dry mixture. Toss in the berries to cover.
2. In another container, mix the cream with the eggs, molasses, and almond milk.
3. Slowly, combine the fixings to make the dough, adding flour as needed.
4. Divide the dough into halves to form two circles.
5. Slice each dough circle into six triangles and bake for about 15 to 20 minutes at 375° Fahrenheit.
6. Leave them in the pan for about 15 minutes to cool. At that time, transfer onto a rack to thoroughly cool.
7. Drizzle with the glaze before serving. Besides, it is also keto-friendly with only four net carbs!

Carrot Cake

Yields Provided: 16
Total Time: 40-45 minutes

Ingredients Required:

- Almond flour (1.5 cups)
- Coconut flour (.5 cup)
- Baking soda (2 tsp.)
- Ground nutmeg (.5 tsp.)
- Baking powder (.5 tsp.)
- Cinnamon (1.5 tsp.)
- Allspice or ginger (.25 tsp.)
- Coconut oil (1 cup)
- Large eggs (4)
- Vanilla extract (2 tsp.)
- Monk fruit sweetener (.75 to 1 cup)
- Packed grated zucchini (1 medium/1.5 cups)
- Loosely packed grated carrots (1 cup - 1 large)
- *Optional*: Walnuts (.5 cup)

  The Frosting:
- Cream cheese (16 oz.)
- Butter (.5 cup or 1 stick)
- Vanilla extract (2 tsp.)
- Powdered monk fruit sweetener (1 cup) or (2 cups) regular powdered sweetener
- Heavy whipping cream (2 tbsp.)
- *Also Needed*: 2 9-inch cake pans

Preparation Technique:

1. Set the oven at 350° Fahrenheit.
2. Prepare the cake pans with a layer of parchment paper.
3. Whisk the almond flour, baking soda, coconut flour, baking powder, nutmeg, cinnamon, and allspice (or ginger) in a mixing container. Set it aside for now.
4. Beat the coconut oil with the eggs and vanilla extract. Stir in the carrots, zucchini, and sweetener. Mix in the flour

mixture and stir until well combined. Fold in the walnuts, as desired.
5. Spread the mixture into the two cake pans.
6. Bake them until browned on top, and the cake is firm to the touch (25-30 min.).
7. Remove from the oven and cool before frosting.
8. Lastly, prepare the frosting. Cream together the butter and cream cheese using an electric mixer. Add powdered sweetener and beat until smooth.
9. Beat in the vanilla extract and heavy whipping cream until light and fluffy.
10. Decorate the cake and serve.

Chocolate Chip GF Mug Cake

Yields Provided: 2
Total Time: 8-10 minutes

Ingredients Required:

- Coconut flour (1.5 tbsp.)
- Baking powder - Viva naturals - ex. (.5 tsp.)
- Cacao powder (2 tbsp.)
- Erythritol powdered sweetener (2 tbsp.)
- Egg (1 medium)
- Double/heavy cream (5 tbsp.)
- Sugar-free chocolate chips (2 tbsp.)
- *Optional:* Vanilla extract (.25 tsp.)

Preparation Technique:

1. Combine each of the dry fixings (baking powder, cacao powder, and sweetener).
2. Fold in the wet fixings (cream, egg, and vanilla extract).
3. Fold in the chocolate chips and let the batter rest for a minute.
4. Melt .5 tsp. of the butter into the two containers (30 seconds).
5. Grease the insides of the two containers. Divide the batter between the containers.
6. Microwave them on high for 1.5 minutes (no longer or the cakes will become dry).
7. Enjoy straight out of the ramekin or turn it out onto a plate.

Cinnamon Bread

Yields Provided: 12
Total Time: 1 hour 20 minutes

Ingredients Required:

Cinnamon Mix:
- Pyure all-purpose (1 tbsp.)
- Cinnamon (1 tsp.)

Bread Batter:
- *Almond flour (2/3 cup)*
- Salt (.5 tsp.)
- Coconut flour (1/3 cup)
- Xanthan gum (.5 tsp.)
- Stevia extract powder (.25 tsp.)
- Baking powder (1 tsp.)
- Pyure all-purpose sweetener (.5 cup)
- Cinnamon (.5 tsp.)
- Butter melted (.5 cup)
- Coconut oil - liquified (3 tbsp.)
- Large eggs (7)
- Vanilla extract (1 tsp.)
- *Also Needed*: 5x9 loaf pan & parchment baking paper/splash of oil

Preparation Technique:

1. Warm the oven to 350° Fahrenheit.
2. Prepare the pan for baking.
3. Mix one tablespoon each of the sweetener and cinnamon in a small mixing container. Set to the side for now.
4. In another container, whisk the dry fixings (xanthan gum, almond flour, coconut flour, stevia, salt, baking powder, erythritol, and cinnamon). Set aside.
5. Toss the eggs, butter, vanilla extract, and coconut oil into a food processor. Pulse until incorporated. Mix with the dry fixings to form the dough.

6. Remove .5 cup of the dough batter and mix into the cinnamon sweetener mix. Set it to the side for now.
7. Pour about half of the batter into the pan. Spoon half of the cinnamon mixture over the batter.
8. Dump the remainder of the plain batter over the cinnamon mixture.
9. Spread the rest of the cinnamon mixture on top. Use a knife to make pretty swirls.
10. Bake for 40 minutes.
11. Lower the heat setting to 325° Fahrenheit.
12. Bake for 15 minutes. (If it's browning too quickly, just tent with a sheet of aluminum foil.)
13. If it's still soft in the center, let it remain in the oven for 5 to 10 minutes. Test for doneness using a cake tester or toothpick.

German Chocolate Cake Made With Zucchini

Yields Provided: 16
Total Time: 50-55 minutes

Ingredients Required:

The Cake:
- Coconut flour (.5 cup)
- Cocoa powder (.5 cup unsweetened)
- Baking powder (1 tsp.)
- Pyure sweetener (.5 cup)
- Ground cinnamon (.5 tsp.)
- Baking soda (1 tsp.)
- Salt (.25 tsp.)
- Coconut oil liquified (.25 cup)
- Eggs (4 large)
- Vanilla (1 tsp.)
- Zucchini (2 cups - shredded)
- Optional: Sugar-free chocolate chips (.5 cup)

The Frosting:
- Unsweetened almond milk (.5 cup)
- Swerve Confectioners Powder (.5 cup)
- Egg (1 yolk)
- Butter or vegan margarine (.25 cup)
- Xanthan gum optional (.25 tsp.)
- Vanilla extract (.5 tsp.)
- Unsweetened shredded coconut (.75 cup)
- Chopped pecans (.5 cup)
- *Also Needed:* 9 by 9 baking pan

Preparation Technique:

1. Set the oven at 350° Fahrenheit.
2. Grease the baking pan. Whisk or sift the flour, cinnamon, cocoa, baking soda, sweetener, salt, and baking powder.
3. Mix in the oil, vanilla, and eggs until incorporated. Stir in the chocolate chips and shredded zucchini.
4. Dump the mixture into the greased pan. Bake it for about 40 minutes.

5. Prepare the frosting. Mix the almond milk with the egg yolk, sweetener, and butter using medium heat in a saucepan. Once the bubbles form, mix in the xanthan gum. Continue heating until thickened.
6. Transfer the pan to the countertop. Stir in the vanilla, coconut, and pecans.
7. Spread the frosting over the cooled cake.

Sugar-Free Donuts

Yields Provided: 9
Total Time: 40-45 minutes

Ingredients Required:

The Donuts:
- Almond flour (1 - 1/3 cups)
- Coconut flour (2/3 cup)
- Baking powder (2 tsp.)
- Low-carb sweetener (.75 cup)
- Salt (1 tsp.)
- Xanthan gum (.5 tsp. or as needed)
- Melted butter or coconut oil (1 tbsp.)
- Large eggs (4 beaten)
- Almond milk or other low-carb milk (.75 cup)
- Vanilla extract (1 tsp.)
- Nutmeg (.25 tsp.)
- Cinnamon (.25 tsp.)

The Frosting:
- Unsweetened almond milk (2 tbsp.)
- Vanilla extract (.5 tsp.)
- Powdered low carb sweetener (.5 cup)
- Liquid stevia (4 drops)

Preparation Technique:

1. Set the oven to 325° Fahrenheit.
2. Grease the donut pan well.
3. Whisk each of the flours with the baking powder, sweetener, xanthan gum, and salt.
4. Fold in the eggs, butter, almond milk, nutmeg, vanilla, and cinnamon. Beat until well blended and empty into the molds (⅔ full).
5. Bake for 18 to 20 minutes. Cool in the pan for about 15 minutes.
6. Prepare and spread the frosting onto the donut tops or dip into a mixture of sweetener and cinnamon.

Cookies

Almond Flour Cookies With Walnuts & Cranberries

Yields Provided: 34 cookies
Total Time: 20-25 minutes

Ingredients Required:

- Almond flour (1.5 cups)
- Cinnamon (.5 tsp.)
- Butter (.5 cup)
- White sweetener - or Swerve or erythritol (.75 cup)
- Large egg (1)
- Sugar-free dried cranberries (1/3 cup)
- Chopped walnuts (.25 cup)

Preparation Technique:

1. Set the oven temperature at 350° Fahrenheit.
2. Transfer the butter and egg to the countertop to become room temperature.
3. Combine almond flour and cinnamon in a mixing container.
4. Cream the sweetener with the butter using an electric mixer. Blend in the egg and slowly stir in the almond flour mixture.
5. Fold in the nuts and cranberries.
6. Scoop the dough onto silicone lined cookie sheets or parchment paper.
7. Bake until the edges are browned (12 to 15 min.).

Chocolate Zucchini Cookies

Yields Provided: 12
Total Time: 30-35 minutes

Ingredients Required:

- Grated zucchini (1 cup)
- Almond flour (1 cup)
- Baking soda (.5 tsp.)
- Coconut flour (.25 cup)
- Cacao powder or unsweetened cocoa powder (.25 cup)
- Salt (.5 tsp.)
- Cinnamon (.25 tsp.)
- Monk fruit sweetener or raw honey (.5 cup)
- Butter flavored coconut oil or ghee (1/3 cup)
- Vanilla extract (1 tsp.)
- Large egg yolk (1)
- Sugar-free chocolate chips or dark chocolate pieces - optional (.25 cup)

Preparation Technique:

1. Prepare the zucchini and wrap in a towel and squeeze out the excess liquid.
2. Whisk the dry fixings (almond flour, cacao powder, salt, baking soda, coconut flour, and cinnamon). Put it to the side for now.
3. In a glass mixing bowl, melt the coconut oil/ghee.
4. Whisk in the sweetener, egg yolk, and vanilla extract.
5. Stir the zucchini into the sweetened mixture and combine it with the dry ingredients. Fold in chocolate if using.
6. Shape the dough tbsp.-sized balls by rolling in your hands.
7. Flatten each ball out and top each with a few pieces of chocolate.
8. Bake the cookies at 350° Fahrenheit for 10 to 12 minutes.

Coconut Chocolate Chip Cookies

Yields Provided: 42 cookies
Total Time: 25 minutes

Ingredients Required:

- Butter (.5 cup)
- Powdered erythritol (.75 cup)
- Stevia (.25 tsp.)
- Polydextrose - optional (.25 cup)
- Blackstrap molasses - optional (1 tsp.)
- Large eggs (4)
- Vanilla extract - sugar-free (1 tsp.)
- Coconut flour sifted (.5 cup)
- Salt (.5 tsp.)
- Unsweetened coconut flaked/grated (2 cups)
- *Optional:* Sugar-free chocolate chips (.5 cup)

Preparation Technique:

1. Grease a baking tin and warm up the oven to reach 350° Fahrenheit. Cream together the butter, erythritol, stevia, molasses, and polydextrose. Whisk and add in the eggs and vanilla.
2. Toss in the salt, coconut flour, and chocolate chips.
3. Drop using a teaspoon-sized mound of cookie dough about one inch apart onto the cookie sheet.
4. Bake the cookies for 12 to 15 minutes. Remove them from the cookie sheet immediately.
5. Cool and store or enjoy now.

Coconut Flour Cranberry Orange Cookies

Yields Provided: 36 cookies
Total Time: 20-25 minutes

Ingredients Required:

- Monk fruit sweetener (.75 cup)
- Butter - softened (.75 cup)
- Eggs (3)
- Baking powder (1.5 tsp.)
- Coconut flour (.5 cup)
- Baking soda (.25 tsp.)
- Dried cranberries - Sugar-free (.25 cup)
- Macadamia nuts chopped (.5 cup)
- Dried grated orange zest (1.5 tsp.)

Preparation Technique:

1. Warm the oven to reach 350° Fahrenheit.
2. Combine the sweetener with the butter and eggs until well incorporated.
3. Sift and blend in the baking powder, coconut flour, and baking soda using the low-speed setting of an electric mixer until well combined.
4. Fold in the orange zest with the cranberries and nuts.
5. Shape into rounds and arrange on the cookie sheet about one inch apart using a parchment or silicone lined cookie sheet.
6. Press down slightly with your fingers to flatten.
7. Bake them for eight to ten minutes. Cool for a few minutes before serving.
8. Enjoy them right out of the fridge or freeze to enjoy later.

Coconut Macaroons

Yields Provided: 40 cookies/20 servings
Total Time: 20-25 minutes

Ingredients Required:

- Water (1/3 cup)
- Monk Fruit sweetener or (.75 cup or less to taste)
- Sea salt (.25 tsp.)
- Sugar-free vanilla extract (.75 tsp.)
- Eggs (2 large)
- Unsweetened shredded coconut (3-4 cups or more as desired)
- *Optional:* Sugar-free chocolate chips

Preparation Technique:

1. Set the oven setting to 350° Fahrenheit.
2. Lightly spray a cookie tin with a spritz of cooking oil spray.
3. In a small saucepan, pour in the water and the sweetener, salt, and vanilla extract. Bring to a boil using the med-high heat temperature setting. Stir and remove from the heat.
4. Use a food processor to combine the egg and coconut flakes. Pour in the syrup and process to form the dough. Using a cookie scoop, place mounds about an inch apart onto the cookie sheet.
5. Bake for eight minutes, and rotate the baking pan in the oven.
6. Bake until lightly browned or for an additional four minutes.
7. Cool on a rack. Drizzle with melted chocolate to your liking.

Peanut Butter Blossoms - Sugar-Free

Yields Provided: 24 cookies
Total Time: 25-30 minutes

Ingredients Required:

- Sukrin Gold - packed or brown sugar replacement (.5 cup)
- Sukrin Gold Fiber Syrup or another tablespoon of Sukrin Gold (1 tbsp.)
- Natural sugar-free peanut butter or use sun butter (.5 cup)
- Egg (1 large)
- Peanut flour sesame flour for nut allergy (.5 cup)
- Baking soda (.5 tsp.)
- Vanilla extract (.5 tsp.)
- Salt (1 pinch if using unsalted peanut butter)
- Low-carb chocolate kiss drops (24) *or* a few chocolate chips
- *Optional:* Monk fruit low carb sweetener

Preparation Technique:

1. Mix the peanut butter and Sukrin Gold until well blended.
2. Prepare a baking sheet with a mat or layer of parchment baking paper.
3. Whisk and mix in the egg until incorporated. Mix in the remaining fixings until uniform dough forms.
4. Roll the dough into balls and roll in the granulated sweetener if desired.
5. Arrange on the baking tin.
6. Press each cookie ball down to about a .5-inch thickness.
7. Bake at 350° Fahrenheit until the cookies are set, about 7 to 10 minutes.
8. Allow cooling for 5 to 10 minutes.
9. Press a chocolate kiss on top of each warm cookie before serving.

Quick & Easy Mug Cakes

Blueberry Mug Cake

Yields Provided: 2
Total Time: 5-8 minutes

Ingredients Required:

- Almond flour (2 tbsp.)
- Salt (1 dash)
- Coconut flour (1 tbsp.)
- Baking powder (.25 tsp.)
- Fresh/Frozen blueberries (2 tbsp.)
- Melted coconut oil (1 tbsp.)
- Heavy cream (2 tbsp. + 1 tsp.)
- Egg (1)
- Vanilla extract (.25 tsp.)
- Lemon extract (.25 tsp.)
- Low-carb sweetener (1 tbsp.)

Preparation Technique:

1. Lightly grease two ramekins using butter.
2. Whisk both types of flour with the baking powder and salt. Stir in the berries. Set to the side for now.
3. Melt the coconut oil in a microwaveable dish. Stir in the egg, heavy cream, sweetener, and extracts.
4. Whisk in the dry components using a fork until it's incorporated.
5. Dump the batter into the ramekins.
6. Microwave using the high setting for 1.5 to 2 minutes (2 minutes in a 900-watt microwave).
7. Serve.

Chocolate Brownie Mug Cake

Yields Provided: 2
Total Time: 4-5 minutes

Ingredients Required:

- Butter (2 tbsp.)
- Almond flour (3 tbsp.)
- Salt (1 pinch)
- Coconut flour (1 tsp.)
- Granulated sugar substitute (1.5 tbsp.)
- Baking powder (.5 tsp.)
- Vanilla (.25 tsp.)
- Egg (1)
- Unsweetened cocoa powder (1 tbsp.)
- Lindt 90% chocolate (1 square - chopped)
- Chopped pecans (optional - 2 tbsp.)

Preparation Technique:

1. Grease two mugs or ramekins.
2. Melt the butter in a bowl (about 30 seconds in the microwave).
3. Add the rest of the fixings. Stir well to combine.
4. Pour the batter into the chosen containers. Microwave them for one minute. Check it, and cook 30 more seconds if needed.
5. Serve with a serving of sugar-free vanilla ice cream or whipped cream.

Coconut Flour Pumpkin Mug Cake

Yields Provided: 2
Total Time: 5 minutes

Ingredients Required:

- Coconut flour (2 tbsp.)
- Egg (1 beaten)
- Pumpkin puree (2 tbsp.)
- Baking powder (.25 tsp.)
- SweetLeaf stevia drops (.25 tsp.)
- Vanilla extract (.5 tsp.)
- Pumpkin pie spice (.5 tsp.)

Preparation Technique:

1. Place each of the fixings into a coffee cup or ramekin.
2. Blend well with a fork.
3. Microwave using the high heat setting for about 1.5 minutes.
4. Remove from the container, if desired.
5. Serve warm with whipped topping.

Vanilla Berry Mug Cake

Yields Provided: 1
Total Time: 5-6 minutes

Ingredients Required:

- Melted butter (1 tbsp.)
- Full-fat cream cheese (2 tbsp.)
- Coconut flour (2 tbsp.)
- Swerve granulated sweetener (1 tbsp. or more to taste)
- Vanilla extract (1 tsp.)
- Baking powder (.25 tsp.)
- Egg (1 medium)
- Frozen raspberries (6)

Preparation Technique:

1. Measure and add the butter and cream cheese in your chosen mug. Microwave it on high for 20 seconds.
2. Whisk the sweetener, coconut flour, vanilla, and baking powder. Mix well. Add the egg. Mix again
3. Scrape down the sides of the mug. Press in six frozen raspberries into the cake batter.
4. Microwave it on high for 1:20 minutes.

Conclusion

I hope you have enjoyed the recipes in the *Gluten Free Cookbook*. I hope it was informative and provided you with all of the tools you need to achieve your goals, whatever they may be. The next step is to gather your shopping list and head to the market.

Try not to become overwhelmed as you challenge yourself to a new gluten-free diet. It will take some time since it seems you are surrounded daily with gluten foods. Your body will not change overnight, and it could take up to six months to become adjusted to the changes.

Remain focused and concentrate on the foods you have every day. Stay on track and leave the junk foods behind. Use some of the delicious recipes provided in your new *Gluten Free Cookbook for Beginners*.

Before you become stressed out, contact a local support group that can be found all over the country. Once you've found a support group, go to their meetings, and associate with individuals who follow the gluten-free diet.

Continue researching the diet plan and rely on recipes such as those you have found in this book. Save money by watching your local sales to acquire ingredients in bulk - if possible. And Always; Check those labels!

Finally, if you found this book useful in any way, a review on Amazon is always appreciated!

Printed by Amazon Italia Logistica S.r.l.
Torrazza Piemonte (TO), Italy